Get Healthy For Your Next 100 Years

by Keith Scott-Mumby MD, PhD

COPYRIGHT

Copyright © 2008 by Keith Scott-Mumby, Scott-Mumby Author Services,

6180 Lake Geneva Dr, Reno, NV 89511, USA.

Dr Keith Scott-Mumby asserts the moral right to be identified as the author of this work.

All rights reserved. No part of this publication may be adapted or reproduced, stored in a retrieval system, or transmitted, in any form or by any means, electronic, mechanical, photocopying, recording or otherwise, without the prior permission of the author and publisher.

This information is provided as information only and may not be construed as medical advice or instruction. No action should be taken based solely on the contents of this publication. Readers should consult appropriate health professionals on any matter relating to their health and well-being.

The publisher shall not be responsible for errors or omissions.

Important Disclaimer

All content within this book is commentary or opinion and is protected under Free Speech laws in all the civilized world. The information herein is provided for educational and entertainment purposes only. It is not intended as a substitute for professional advice of any kind. Dr. Keith Scott-Mumby MD, PhD assumes no responsibility for the use or misuse of this material.

Therefore no warranty of any kind, whether expressed or implied, is given in relation to this information or any of the external services referred to. This is a comprehensive limitation of liability that applies to all damages of any kind, including (without limitation) compensatory; direct, indirect or consequential damages; loss of data, income or profit; loss of or damage to property and claims of third parties. Neither shall Professor Scott-Mumby be liable for any content of any external internet sites listed and services listed.

The statements made about products and services have not been evaluated by the U.S. Food and Drug Administration. They are not intended to diagnose, treat, cure, or prevent any condition or disease.

Always consult your own licensed medical practitioner if you are in any way concerned about your health. You must satisfy yourself of the validity of the professional qualifications of any health care provider you contact as a result of this book.

If you cannot agree to these terms, destroy the book if you downloaded it free, or ask for a refund and then destroy it, if payment was made.

These are serious issues and intense pressure often falls on publishers of such needed information, from parties who do not wish you to know anything other than what they tell you is true. We ask you not to create problems by irresponsible use or spread of this valuable information.

All trademarks, registered trademarks and service marks mentioned in the book are the property of their respective owners.

Disclaimer

Please understand when I suggest a particular product or service may be beneficial that I cannot be responsible for what happens if you use the product or submit to the service. Everyone is different and variable responses and tolerance to substances, even those from natural sources, is one of the mainstays of my teachings.

All my suggestions are made in good faith and in the knowledge that they are well tolerated by the majority of individuals and effective in most cases.

—Keith Scott-Mumby MD, MB ChB, PhD

Dr. Keith special insights

Quotes On Aging...

"The soul is born old but grows young. That is the comedy of life. And the body is born young and grows old. That is life's tragedy."
- Oscar Wilde

"The age of a woman doesn't mean a thing. The best tunes are played on the oldest fiddles."
- Ralph Waldo Emerson

"We don't stop playing because we grow old; we grow old because we stop playing."
- George Bernard Shaw

"Age is an issue of mind over matter. If you don't mind, it doesn't matter."
- Mark Twain

"Age is not a particularly interesting subject. Anyone can get old. All you have to do is live long enough."
- Groucho Marx

"I don't believe one grows older. I think that what happens early on in life is that at a certain age one stands still and stagnates."
- T. S. Eliot

"There is a fountain of youth: it is your mind, your talents, the creativity you bring to your life and the lives of people you love. When you learn to tap this source, you will truly have defeated age."
- Sophia Loren

"Old age isn't so bad; when you consider the alternatives."
- Maurice Chevalier

...More Quotes On Aging

"Old age ain't no place for sissies."
- Henry Louis Mencken

"Old age is not a disease - it is strength and survivorship, triumph over all kinds of vicissitudes and disappointments, trials and illnesses."
- Maggie Kuhn

"Grow old along with me! The best is yet to be, the last of life, for which the first was made. Our times are in his hand who saith, 'A whole I planned, youth shows but half; Trust God: See all, nor be afraid!'"
- Robert Browning

"Men of age object too much, consult too long, adventure too little, repent too soon, and seldom drive business home to the full period, but content themselves with a mediocrity of success."
- Dale Carnegie

"Anyone who stops learning is old, whether at twenty or eighty. Anyone who keeps learning stays young. The greatest thing in life is to keep your mind young."
- Henry Ford

Contents

The Magic Of Aging! / 1

Introduction / 5
Do You Want To Be A Crock Or A Classic Car? 5
Survival Probability 7
Life Span and Life Expectancy 8
National Geographic Survey 9
#1. We Don't Die Of Age, We Die Of Disease 10
    Regeneration 11
#2. Live a Younger Life 11
    Preserve Your Health Coupons 12
    So where is all this leading? 12
    Science To The Rescue 13
#3. Destructive vs. Constructive Metabolism 14
#4. A Note on Dying 15
    Avoiding the Speed Bumps! 15
    Statistics Can Lie 16
    How Many Bumps Did You Say? 16
    Doctors Are the Number One Killers 17
    Cancer and Heart Disease 17

What Exactly Is Aging? Anti-Aging Models / 19
Oxidative Damage Model 19
Genes Model 20
Carbohydrate Control Model (Insulin Resistance) 22
Telomeres and DNA Damage Model 22
    Hot Off the Press 23
    Help Your Telomeres 24
Stress Model 24
    Killer Cortisol 24
Inflammation Model 25
Sources of Inflammation 26
The Hayflick Limit 27
Attitude is Crucial 27

Emotional Longevity / 29

- Thoughts and Actions ... 30
- Environment and Relationships ... 30
- Personal Achievement and Equality ... 31
- Emotions and Stress ... 32
  - Emotions and Survival ... 32
  - Loneliness ... 32
  - The Heart and Negative Emotions ... 33
  - Control Over Your Life Status vs. Stress ... 33
  - My Advice ... 34
  - "Yes" Can Seriously Hurt You ... 35
- The Power Of NO ... 35
- Faith and Meaning ... 38

Quench Inflammation / 41

- Inappropriate Inflammation ... 41
- How Do You Rate? ... 42
- Inflammatory Markers ... 43
  - The Missing Link Between Belly Fat and Heart Disease ... 44
  - Drugs for Inflammation? ... 45
  - Pioglitazone ... 46
  - My Own Contributions ... 46
  - Stealth Pathogens ... 47
  - How Do We Get Rid Of Stealth Pathogens? ... 48
  - The Matrix In Health And Disease ... 48
  - Deep Tissue Cleansing ... 48
  - Remedy Mixtures ... 49
  - Triatomic Oxygen ... 50
  - Insufflation ... 51
  - Prostaglandins ... 52

Your Personal Survival Diet / 55

- How To Live 100 Years ... 55
  - It worked ... 56
- Inflammatory Foods ... 56
- Personalized Nutrigenomics ... 58
- SNPs (pronounced "snips") ... 59
  - Example: Let's Look at Codeine ... 59
- Vitamins Alter Gene Expression ... 60

Food Pharmaceuticals 60
What's wrong with the "bad gene" theory? 60

Carbohydrate Control / 63

Are You Serious About Staying Out Of A Nursing Home For Your Last 20 Years On Earth? 63
Low Carbs Help Weight Control 64
    What should you do? 65
    Are You At Risk? 65
    A Big Bum Protects! 66
    Obesity 66
    Metabolic Syndrome 67
Inflammation Again 68
Diabetes 68
    Laboratory Testing 69
    What You Can Do 70
    Supplements 71
    Fiber 71
    Products 72

Detox - Stemming the chemical blizzard / 73

Human Chemical Contamination 73
The Liver 74
Understanding Detox Pathways 75
Toxic Intermediates 76
Phase 3 77
What To Do 77
    Step 1 - Seek A Competent Health Specialist 77
    Step 2 - Get Rid Of Ongoing Sources 78
    Step 3 - Clean Up Your Environment 78
    Step 4 - Improve Your Diet, Get Rid Of Toxic Foods 79
    4. Drink Enough Water To Help Your Kidneys 79
    Saunas 79

Nutritional Supplements Against Aging / 81

My Top 12 *Non-Hormonal* Anti-Aging Supplements 81
    1. L-Carnosine 81
    2. Trimethyl Glycine (TMG) 81
    3. Gingko Biloba 82

- 4. S-ADENOSYL METHIONINE (SAMe, pronounced Sammy) 82
- 5. N-Acetyl-Cysteine (NAC) 82
- 6. Phosphatidyl Choline (And Phosphatidylserine) 82
- 7. Coenzyme-Q-10 83
- 8. Boron 83
- 9. Alpha-Lipoic Acid 83
- 10. Vitamin E 83
- 11. Vitamin D 84
- 12. Essential Fatty Acids 85
- Iodine, The Orphan Nutrient 87
- Organic vs. Inorganic Iodine 88
- Iodine Loading Test 88

Other Nutritional Supplements 88
CoQ10 Update 89

The Antioxidants Story / 91

Oxygen Is A Poison! 91
- Definitions 91

Respiration 92
- Reactive Oxygen Species 92

Anti-Oxidants 93
The Ultimate Anti-Ager Of All 94
Also Rans 95
Glutathione, The True Miracle 96
Surprise Anti-Oxidant! 96
Attacks On Anti-Oxidants 97
Polyphenols, Poly What? 98
Green Tea's Powerful Antioxidants 98
Ashwagandha 99
Lutein, Zeazanthin and Macular Degeneration 100
ORAC Values, What Do They Mean? 101
- How The Food Is Prepared 101

Chocolate 102
The Science 103

Hormones, The Good, The Bad, The Ugly / 107

Superhormones Outside The Box 107
Growth Hormone: Who Needs It? 108
- What You Can Do 109

Secretogogues..110
Men's Stuff..**111**
　　　Testosterone Supplements 112
　　　CAUTION Aromataze 112
Vitamin K and prostate..**113**
　　　Which Brings Us To Prostate Health 114
　　　Tossing Away The Risk! 114
Women's Stuff..**115**
　　　We come back to HRT..116
　　　The Miracle Herbal Hormone 116
　　　Side effect or bonus?..117
　　　Authenticity..117
　　　Pregnenolone: The Mother Hormone 118
DHEA **119**
　　　Unwanted Effects 120
　　　7-Keto DHEA 120
Blood And Saliva Tests **121**
　　　For women: 121
　　　For men: 121

Heart And Vascular Health / 123

A New Disease **124**
Blood Pressure is a Killer **126**
The Cholesterol Myth **127**
Dating Your Arteries **128**
The Inflammation Connection **130**
Plaques Are Not Where It Starts **131**
What You Can Do...**131**
Reduce Inflammation at all Costs...**132**
　　　Heart Savers...133
　　　External Counter Pulsation..134
　　　Intravenous Chelation Therapy 134
　　　The Chelation Facts 135
　　　Vitamin K2...135
　　　Vitamin D3. Now Here's a Surprise!..136
　　　Arterial Scurvy...136
　　　Vitamin C and Hypertension 137
　　　Reducing Clotting Tendency..137
　　　Why do You Need to Know?..138

Brain Savers / 139

The Brain and Aging 139
Facts You May Not Know 139
What You Can Do 140
Alzheimer's Disease 140
Risk Factors 141
Diet Changes 142
Treatment For Alzheimer's 143
IV Anti-Oxidant Therapy 144
Brain Saver Supplements 145
Alpha-Lipoic Acid and Acetyl-L-Carnitine 145
Phosphatidyl Choline and Serine 146
Gotu Kola 146
Ginkgo Biloba 146
Ginseng 146
Vinpocetine 147
Other Brain Nutrients 147
Folic Acid Helps Prevent Cognitive Decline 147
Hormones and Brain Function 148
More Supplements With Specific Mood-Boosting Benefits 148
Phenylalanine 149
S-Adenosyl methionine (SAMe) 149
Tryptophan and 5-hydroxytryptophan (5HT) 149
Carnitine 151

Look After Your Skin / 153

Diet 153
Wine Is Good! 154
If You Can't Drink Alcohol, Eat Chocolate! 155
Botox 155
Homeopathic Botox (Better!) 156
Chelation 156
Hyaluronic Acid (Ha) 157
Skin Creams And Unguents 157
Enter Al Sears MD 158
What Not To Allow On Your Skin 159
Telomeres Breakthrough for Skin Aging 160
SCENAR Cosmetology Technique 161
Star Trek Medicine 162

Movement and Exercise / 163

- Take It Easy! 163
- I Bet Nobody Told You That Before! But It's True. 163
- Eight Scientific Studies Show Why Not To Exercize Hard 164
- Being a Couch Potato is Bad! 166
- Do You Have Sitting Disease? 166
- How Much Is Good? 167
- Have You Heard Of Fit And Fat? It's A Myth! 168
    - Posture 169
    - Dance 170
    - Yoga 171
    - Tai Chi & Qigong 172
    - Exercise Sleep Crossover 172
    - Osteoporosis and Bone Strength 173
    - Hormone Therapy 173
    - Bone Densitometry 175
    - Nutritional Factors Affecting Bone Strength 175
    - Magnesium 175
    - Folic Acid 176
    - Boron 176
    - Strontium 176
    - Other Important Nutrients 176
    - Non-Nutritional Factors 177

Miscellaneous Factors / 179

- Sleep and Vitality 179
    - Is There A Causative Link? 181
- Coffee an Anti-Ager? 181
    - Anti-Inflammatory? 182
    - Hmmm. That Dreamy Smell… 182
- Enjoy a Glass of Red Wine! 183
    - Defining Drinking Levels 184
    - Resveratrol 185
    - The Real Demon in Drink 186
    - A Few Figures 187
    - Caution 188
- The Dangers in Your Mouth 189
    - Dental hygiene 189
- Heavy Metal Poisoning 190
    - Heavy Metals and Cancer 190

  Avoiding Heavy Metal Exposure is Impossible 191
  Sources of Heavy Metal 191
  Persistence in the environment 193
  Protection From Other Metals 193
  What Can You Do? 193
Chelation **194**
Laughter And Play **195**

Love And Sex / 197
Vitamin L 197
What Can You Do? 198
  Remember, you get back what you give out. 199
  Just do it! 199
  That Loving Touch 199
  Women Are The Health Sentries 200
  Love is the Key 201
Sex Matters 201
  Sex Releases Stress 202
  The Midlife Crisis 203
  Characteristics Of The Andropause 203
  The True Mid-Life Crisis 204
  What Lies Beyond 204
  Women 205
  What You Can Do 205
Pueraria mirifica, a herbal remedy from Thailand,
Herbal Remedy From Thailand 206
  The Problem 207
  Selective Estrogen Receptor Modulators (SERMs) 207
  Men Too! 207
Reversing Aging 208
  Dosage and Sources 208
  Sum Up Properties Of Pueraria Mirifica 209

Engine Speed. The Thyroid Gland. / 211
Immunity 212
Accelerating Problem 212
The Broda Barnes Temperature Test 213
Other Tests 213
Treatment 213
Synthetic vs. Natural Replacement 214

Pseudo-Science 214
Suppliers 215
Good website for self-help information and notes: 216

Electromagnetic Energy Devices That May Help Prevent Aging / 217

Pulsed Electromagnetic Devices For Extra Longevity 217
General Health Benefits 218
PEMF To The Rescue 219
Let There Be Light! 221
Seeing Red 221
Cytochrome Oxidase 223
Red Light Right Up Your Nose 223
Far Infrared Light 224
Light Helmets 225

Your Personal Anti-Aging Program / 227

The Magic Of Aging!

Yes, magic. It's a wondrous process that has more positives than negatives. Middle age and beyond is not something most species get to live through. New scientific ideas suggest that this vital later phase of life is precisely why human beings have ended up taking over the planet!

If you are over 50, pat yourself on the back for being Nature's most highly evolved organism. Biologically and socially, you are streets ahead of the youngsters who hog today's limelight!

But why did evolution take us down that path? The answer is inextricably bound up with the exceptional nature of humans. We are a brilliantly adaptive species, for which the process of learning has been crucial. Today we can read books and Google information. But before the advent of writing, much less computers, skills had to be learned and it took time; decades in fact.

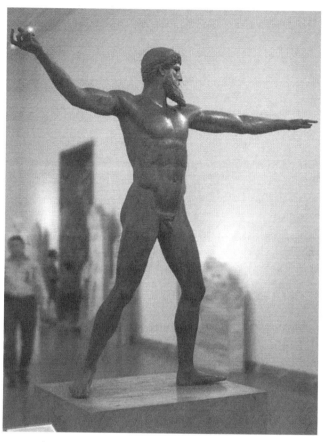

Oftentimes, the necessary skills were not accumulated till after the age of 40. Surviving long enough to acquire these skills would be a strong evolutionary advantage, which would be selected for by Nature.

These skills would be passed on to other members of the tribe and that would give them the advantage over competitors, whether the human kind of the sabre-toothed kind! We would quickly "develop" a middle age, even if we didn't start with one.

Middle age would be a valuable commodity that Nature chose for us!

Important changes take place in middle age which, although we resist them, do seem to have positive qualities. Most body systems deteriorate very little during this stage of life. We just start to look different (not true of most species). But the mind could be stronger, not weaker.

This came home to me vividly one day in the National Archeological Museum at Athens. I was looking at a magnificent bronze of a Poseidon (Neptune), carrying a spear. Presumably he was considered a god because he was smart? He had hard abs and a flat belly, he looked lean, fit and mean; then it struck me… This "god" was in his forties, possibly fifties!

So: to carry out their roles in society, middle-aged people need not necessarily think better or worse than younger adults, but they may have learned to think differently. Indeed, functional brain imaging studies suggest that they sometimes use different brain regions than young people when performing the same tasks, raising the possibility that the nature of thought itself changes as we get older.

But it's a slow change. You can see it just by looking at older people: they are barely different in their thoughts and attitudes, just because their skin has gone wrinkly, they now need glasses and they have a pot belly! Only right at the very end do we tend to slide down the slope of decay.

Even that may be abnormal. There is still heated debate over whether the proportion of the population who lose mental function are really part of the normal spectrum or whether they had a disease process running, leading to the decay that we call senescence. The alert mental faculties seen in extreme old-age individuals, some of them beyond 120 years of age, suggests that any degree of mental decline is pathological, rather than "normal".

Again, you only have to look to begin realizing that older people are actually evolved—developed, if you like. They are, well… wiser! In many ways they are fitter to survive than youngsters, who do not have the survival skills that the elders have learned over the years.

The evolved mature adult, which we call middle-aged, may be just about the most advanced thing existing on the planet! That creature is so full of knowledge and skills that he or she is able to conquer the environment.

Middle-aged and wise individuals may be the very reason Mankind has become such a successful species. Collectively, older people have developed, held and transmitted the knowledge that has enabled us to survive and flourish as a species, by cleverly learning to extract resources which are beyond the reach of most other animals, so giving us the edge.

This supposes that in the past many adults have reached middle age. But isn't it true that most primitive societies lead lives that are short, nasty and brutish, as Thomas Hobbes said?

Actually, that's a misconception. True, in times past, life expectancy was appallingly short by today's standard: 35 or less, compared the today's value of around 75 years or more. But that was almost entirely due to the high infant mortality.

Once past the danger zone, as it were, then adults, even in Stone Age times, tended to live untill middle age and beyond. Archeological pre-history records make that clear; older folks abounded. When we reach documented history, then it is discovered that adults could survive till their eighth or ninth decade.

Even in Ancient Greece, making it to 90 or 100 was not amazing. Democritus is said to have lived to over 100; Xenophanes of Colophon and Eratosthenes of Cirene, to 95 years; and Pyrrho of Ellis, to 90. This was long before antibiotics and low cholesterol diets!

Epimenides of Crete (7th, 6th centuries BC), was said to have lived 154, 157 or even 290 years. Do not dismiss such an idea. You will read in this amazing book that we already have the mechanisms, without modern science, to live to 300 years on average.

So middle and old age has always been around. I have hinted it is valuable, to the individual and to the tribe. Maybe we have evolved a middle age period, which is not shared by other species?

In prehistory, and still today, human survival is entirely dependent on skilled gathering of rare, valuable resources. Humans cooperate, plan and innovate so they can extract what they need from their environment - be that roots to eat, hides to wear or rare metals to coat smartphone touchscreens. We lead an energy-intensive, communication-driven, information-rich way of life, and it was the evolution of middle age which supported this.

For example, hunter-gatherer societies often have complex and difficult techniques for finding and processing food that take a long time to learn. There is evidence that many hunter-gatherers (which is what we humans really are) take decades to learn their craft and resource-acquiring abilities may not peak until they are over 40.

Gathering sufficient calories is crucial for the success of a human community, especially since young humans take so long to grow up. Our children are virtually parasites for their first 10 to 14 years.

Research suggests that a human child requires resources to be provided by multiple adults - almost certainly more than two young parents. For example, a recent study of two groups of South American hunter-gatherers suggested that each couple requires the help of an additional 1.3 non-reproducing adults to provide for their children (Proceedings of the Royal Society B, vol 276, p 1674).

Thus, middle-aged people may be seen as an essential human innovation, an elite caste of skilled, experienced "super-providers" on which the rest of us depend.

The other key role of middle age is the propagation of information. We are born knowing and being able to do almost nothing. Each of us depends on a continuous infusion of skills, knowledge and customs - collectively known as culture - if we are to survive. And the main route by which culture is transferred is by middle-aged people showing and telling their children what to do, as well as the young adults with whom they hunt and gather.

So, if you made it this far, give yourself a hearty round of applause. You deserve it, you super-being you!

Introduction

"Youth is wasted on the young," said George Bernard Shaw (1856-1950). Notice he managed to live 94 years and was fit as a butcher's dog until his last day (can you believe he fell out of a tree while pruning it?)

Shaw was always so witty and yet so wise. In fact, a new word was coined for the English language: *Shavian* (after Shaw), meaning acid humor with a lot of truth in it, like the phrase I quoted above.

How right Shaw was. By the time we start to understand the secrets of a good life, our looks have started to decay. At the point when we should be at our wisest, most vibrant and sexiest, our energies are fading fast. Kids don't know what they have and while we watch them squandering it we can only sigh!

But it simply isn't fair! If we could link some of the wisdom we gain over the years to the seemingly inexhaustible energy of the younger generation that would be a formula for a life well lived.

Well, the Boomer generation (and I'm one) have decided we are not going to take this lying down. We want to live to 120, enjoy every minute, look great, work hard, play hard, and have lots of sex and dance on our last day!

In fact, we Boomers have started an anti-aging revolution. When I went through medical school, (and still today in many quarters) medical scientists insisted aging was a process nobody could do anything about it, believing life expectancy was fixed at birth.

What baloney! The first sign people were not aging as they were supposed to was in the women celebrities from the 70s and 80s. Diane Cannon, Elizabeth Taylor, Joan Collins, and Raquel Welch looked terrific at 40! I know I was growing older too and coming up behind them. But just look at their photos from that era. It can't be argued, surely, that women approaching middle age could look really good. Ha me!

Do You Want To Be A Crock Or A Classic Car?
Most people think of anti-aging as living too long and being a crumbly old ruin. "I'd rather die young!" is the cheerful reply. This actually misses the point entirely. There are dozens of degenerative processes, which take place in our bodies and, if unchecked, they cause a progressive inability to function, slow clumsy movements, aches and pains, confused and irrational thinking, wrinkles and unpleasant looking skin, weakness and frailty, stooped posture, incontinence, and other humiliating conditions, which even the heartiest soul will find demeaning.

The sad thing is we are taught to expect these infirmities as "normal." While they are common, that doesn't make them normal. It is one of the prime maxims in my clinic that what would be unhealthy in a young person is unhealthy in someone much older. We work on correcting these factors as completely as possible.

That doesn't mean we can turn back the clock to our youth but it does mean almost all the parameters by which we judge our health and vitality are to some degree controllable and reversible. Being an old crumbly is what happens when you DON'T take care of the anti-aging issues! You don't have to decay as you age.

The truth is our bodies are not static and unchanging. Just like a machine, they face a slow but steady decline, which is what materially oriented doctors like to believe and cling to.

Rather, we are a dynamic integrated system of cells, organs, and fluids, constantly renewing and replacing itself every few months. The heart and brain you have now isn't the one you had last year! Even the old idea that you cannot replace brain cells is proven foolish and a false doctrine.

The real miracle is that life is able to do this at all, working somewhat against the Second Law of Thermodynamics, never mind the cut-off that the process eventually begins to fail.

The medical profession and drug cartels are now showing an intense interest in aging and they spend a huge amount on researching biological repair and regeneration mechanisms, not because they care, but because there is big money potential. As a result, anti-aging science is rapidly advancing, and thousands of articles on age-related topics are published every month.

Aging has causes. You will see it is not pre-programmed. For example, one of the causes of aging is the decline in growth hormone secreted by the pituitary gland, which takes place in later years. Children who produce little or no growth hormone age and die wizened and dwarfed within 10 – 12 years, an unpleasant condition known as progera. Doctors now recognize a growth hormone deficiency syndrome in adults.

According to Dr Silvio Inzucchi "Growth hormone deficiency is now formally recognized as a specific clinical syndrome, typified by decreased muscle mass, increased body fat (predominantly at intra-abdominal sites), decreased exercise capacity, osteopenia, abnormal lipid profiles, and diminished feeling of well-being" (Hospital Practice, Jan 15, 1997). But wait - doesn't that sound like a good description of aging? Osteopenia means thinning of bones and abnormal lipids refers to cholesterol and other blood fats.

If it sounds as if supplementing growth hormone might be the answer to all our problems, it isn't. As you will discover as you read, things are not that simple. It would be like putting high-octane jet fuel in a vehicle, which has not been properly maintained. You might even wreck the engine!

There is no evidence at all that growth hormone supplementation extends length of life, but it could make the quality of life better for some, by restoring lost strength, zest and well-being. This accords well with the main thrust of the anti-aging movement, which does not promise eternal life but rather believes that it's all about enjoying maximum quality of being to the very end. As one patient put it: to die as young as possible but as late as possible.

This is in complete contrast to the ruling dictum of the medical profession as a whole, which is that you must accept aging as an inevitable and uncontrollable process. There is absolutely no scientific validity to the view. It stems entirely from ignorance and prejudice. Instead of awakening to the possibilities of extended health and vigor, which should be the prime aim, doctors continue to peddle the gloomy doctrine of terminal senility. Now a fuller picture is coming into focus, which is very different from the ignorance, confusion, dogma, and rigid thinking of the past.

The timely emergence of the credible science of anti-aging is most welcome. It's great news, because most of it is within each individual's personal control. In this book alone, there are over one thousand key strategies for beating the aging process and enjoying a younger life for longer. You need this knowledge! The fact remains, almost anyone reading this book is likely to live beyond eighty years of age and around half will live beyond their century.

But what do the statistics of aging tell us?

Survival Probability

More and more people are living to a great age. Seventy odd years may be the life expectancy when you are born (varies in each country); but once you have reached retirement age, the average life expectancy goes up to 85 and beyond. That means lots of people are going to live to ninety and beyond.

In the USA, we are now approaching 100,000 individuals who have reached one hundred years of age (Nov 2008) and in the UK, there are 10,000. Figures from other industrialized countries report similar numbers. Moreover, the total of centenarians is rising fast.

The scary thing is that these figures even include the suicidal couch potatoes who overeat, are grossly obese, take no exercise, no rescue supplements, and are entirely ignorant of just how much they are damaging their future with this unnatural lifestyle. I find that remarkable. Something is happening, over and above the Boomer generation, who tend to take care of themselves quite well.

According to the American Academy of Anti-Aging Medicine and the World Health Organization, fully 50% of the post-war "baby boom" generation now in good health will reach the age of 100. There will eventually be millions of individuals over 100 years old. You could be a centenarian, whether you choose to or not.

It's crazy not to prepare for age and try to prevent it being an unpleasant, unhealthy experience - as it is for some, though not, of course, everyone. And this is a key point: if any one person is fit at age 100 years, it means everyone can be.

Growing old does not harm you!

Life Span and Life Expectancy

Average life expectancy and maximum life span should never be confused. Enthusiasts sometimes muddle the two, either unintentionally or with intended blurring of the issues. Average life expectancy figures given above do not tell us how long the longest achievable life span may be. So far, living beyond one hundred and twenty years is rare—but not nearly as rare as you have been hoodwinked into thinking.

The truth is coming at you. Are you ready?

Man is a remarkably long-lived animal. If we examine other mammalian species and multiply their average life expectancy by heart rate, it seems most species get the same few million beats and then it is curtains! However, man has several times this number (over 2 billion).

> **In the USA, we are now approaching 100,000 individuals who have reached one hundred years of age (Nov 2008)**

The longest living mammals appear to be whales and some species are now known to survive over two centuries. There seems no logical reason why we cannot do the same - but be sure to read about the Hayflick limit later in this report.

The oldest well-documented case of extreme old age in humans was Dr Li Ching-Yun, who lived in Western China. His obituary appeared in the New York Times May 8th 1933 and in The Times on May 6th. His age was given as 256 and reading about this case was supposedly what inspired James Hilton to write his Shangri-La classic Lost Horizon.

Records exist showing Li Ching-Yun born in 1677 and the Chinese government he was sent him official certificates at ages 150, 200, and 250, so there is a fair degree of certainty this was correct. At the astonishing age of 250 he lectured medical students in Beijing on the art of living a long and healthy life.

Dr. Li's reported formula was "Keep a quiet heart; sit like a tortoise; sleep like a dog". These accords well with modern anti-aging science, which says, avoid stress, avoid inflammatory over-exertion, and sleep at least 8 hours! Maybe there was surprise wisdom in the 60s maxim "Drop out. Take it easy! Chill out!" It may be significant that the most noticeably long-lived societies, like the Hunzas in the Himalayas, the Georgians in what used to be the USSR and the Vilcabambans in Ecuador are all non-industrial societies with little reason to rush and strive.

If you want to live longer and chill out more, make sure your heart rate slows down. Mine's between 58 and 64 normally, way below the "average" of 72 beats per minute. To get your pulse rate down low you MUST eliminate stressor foods. Swallowing foods that stress your body leads to a continuous overactive heartbeat.

To learn how to eliminate stressor foods is easy. I already wrote a book for you about it, called "Diet Wise". Before that (1950s) Arthur F. Coca MD wrote a great text called "The Pulse Test". It showed the world how to eliminate allergy foods and poorly tolerated foods (which stress the body) by simply counting heart rate after eating sample foods.

His technique was slightly flawed but I added my knowledge and I show you how to get past the phenomenon of refractory foods (the ones that are bad but don't react overtly when you test them). Coca didn't know about this "hidden allergy" effect.

Get a copy of Diet Wise book here: http://www.DietWiseBook.com

If you've got one already and your pulse is still over 75, read it again! You missed some important life-saving data!

National Geographic Survey

A 1970 survey of the Georgian (Caucasus) region showed that 69 individuals out of every 100,000 reached the age one hundred. Yet in the USA, the world's richest and what should be the healthiest nation, that figure is a miserable 3 per 100,000. There is certainly something to learn here from societies that are less wealthy, less organized, and less hectic. It's also the reason to mistrust almost everything you are told by a medical profession considering the longevity figures for America!

National Geographic Magazine, January 1973, carried an interesting article by Alexander Leaf MD about the centenarians of Georgia in the former USSR. At that time the oldest person living was Shirali Mislimov, who was 168 years old and still riding a horse. Unfortunately, the authorities would not allow the scientists to interview him. But the article features a woman called Khfaf Lasuria, who was calculated by visitors to be between 130 and 140 years old.

At the age of 111 she had retired from her work (picking tea) and she was still travelling alone by bus visiting relatives. Her conversation was crisp and lucid, and her memory formidable. Khfaf drank a glass of vodka and smoked a packet of cigarettes every day, which makes you wonder: what does the medical profession really know? Here was a woman defying her age while the best of civilized medicine in the world (supposedly) was letting its people turn into sad incompetent invalids from the sixth decade onwards.

Other striking cases uncovered by Leaf showed centenarian men and women able to work a full day, dance nimbly, ride horses and engage in regular sexual activity. By way of contrast, Leaf himself declared he was exhausted trying to follow Gabriel Chapnian, a man of 117, up a steep hill while he (Chapnian) carried a pail of newly harvested potatoes! And before you ask, yes these were carefully documented ages. This is a Catholic community and baptism records have existed in detail for centuries.

Scientists put their longevity achievements down to low calorie diets; but the individuals themselves were almost uniform in their appraisal of the reason pertaining to lack of stress. One man of 108 told Leaf "I never had a single enemy, I read no books, and have no worries". This attack on literacy appeared more than once in interviews; the same Gabriel Chapnian, asked why Americans died much younger, replied "Too literate!"

Beware then, reading this book may shorten your life! (Just kidding).

#1. We Don't Die Of Age, We Die Of Disease

Anti-aging doctors are united about one thing: we do not die of age we die of diseases. The extreme old age cases you read about did not finally run out of life! They contracted a terminal illness and were whisked away. Nine out of ten times bronchopneumonia was the reason. They made it past the dangers of heart disease, diabetes, and cancer, only to succumb to an everyday infection, which because of their frailty, proved too severe.

The fact is the major killers - heart disease, stroke, diabetes and most cancers are easily preventable if you go about it the right way. The appalling toll of deaths are simply a measure of the incompetence of a medical profession obsessed with drugs and treating only symptoms, instead of taking effective and proven action directed towards the known causes of these conditions.

We need to go further upstream in the health cascade and deal with the true causes behind disease conditions, because trying to eliminate the disease once you have it is much harder to do.

The prestigious journal Science, reported, if we could eliminate heart disease, cancer, stroke, and diabetes as major causes of death, life expectancy would rise to 99.4 years!

Sadly, most people wait until it is too late. The smart ones, who think ahead and plan, will realize anti-aging is not really an option. You have to do it, or suffer unpleasant and maybe unbearable consequences.

It may help to picture this in terms of the aging of a motor car. Typically, a well-used car will last 10- 20 years and then fall apart, becoming too unsafe to be repaired. The better the maintenance, the longer it takes to crumble. If you omit routine oil changes and other essential care, the car will mechanically fail sooner. Yet some of the CLASSIC CARS, which are 80, 90 or even more than 100 years old, are in sweet running order and perform reliably. Why is that? The answer is obvious - it screams at you, **they have been properly looked after.**

It's exactly the same with the human body. You have to ask yourself, do you want to be a classic car or an old "banger", rusting and clanking away? I doubt many would choose to be a banger. Yet that is the mentality of anyone who doesn't begin to take effective care of their health NOW.

We have one proven advantage over mechanical objects. Our bodies can regenerate to a considerable degree. It has been a long-standing medical hoax to tell people they have to put up with miserable health conditions, just because the doctors don't have the cure.

The fact is, almost all disease is reversible. Nature can fix things when given the chance and the right raw materials. To invoke the car comparison once more, think of old rusting hulks that have been salvaged and tenderly nursed back into fine running condition by devoted enthusiasts.

We can do it too!

For answers, turn to nature, rather than the drug industry. There are many exciting ways to gain back your health, even after many years of believing you were stuck with it. You probably already know of people curing themselves of arthritis, cancer, heart disease, and so on, without resorting to any further drastic medical intervention. These results show the way for us all. You can indeed recover your health!

Combine this with the many breakthroughs in anti-aging science, and there is no good reason, other than self-neglect, to accept the breakdown of age. People routinely feel a sense of complete life renewal, increased vigor, mental clarity, and sexual pleasure once they turn back the clock. You can too!

In the words of Dr Walter Pierpaoli and Dr William Regeleson:

"Ours is the first generation that need not experience senescence, the dismal physical decline now associated with old age. We are the first generation that need not resign ourselves to accepting the fate that our later years will be filled with debility and disease. Ours is the first generation that has the capacity, by resetting our aging clocks, to actually prolong youthful health and vitality into our eighties, nineties, and possibly even our hundreds".

Do you want to grow old and sick or live a healthy zestful life to the very end? Do you want to be a classic car or on old crock? It's up to you!

Regeneration

Sure there are possibilities for stopping or slowing the aging process. But there's even better news, because the science of anti-aging says it is possible to turn back the clock.

At the age of 75, you still have 85% of the brain cells you were born with, and the good news is scientists at the Salk Institute in La Jolla, California have proven brain cells can replace themselves. Previously it was thought loss of brain cells was permanent, but we now know we have the potential to regenerate and revitalize our brains.

Add to that the fact we now realize our brains are very plastic (a technical term) and can be shaped and molded. Continuous use of our brains opens up new neural pathways and the synaptic connections, which link our brain cells, can be dramatically increased by daily use.

We'll talk about this more later in the report.

#2. Live a Younger Life

Do you want to live forever? Probably not! But most of us would be reassured to know we would feel fit, well and active right up to the end.

It was Jonathan Swift, author of GULLIVER'S TRAVELS, who first remarked that nobody wants to die; yet nobody wants to grow old either. Can we do anything about the unhappy paradox here?

Well, yes. The new science of anti-aging is not just about living longer, although I am convinced and so are many doctors like me, that if you do the right things you can extend your life considerably. It's more about increasing the quality of life. It's about feeling good, remaining active, keeping your mind alive and alert, staying free from pain and stiffness and continuing with that most important of human feel-good activities… sex.

It's a great paradox of our lives that during the process of striving and achievement, that just as we reach the pinnacle of our careers, the top of the corporate ladder, and social life, biology begins to let us down. Just as we reach the dreams we aspired to, and have the time and the money to fulfill them, we find ourselves facing stroke, heart disease, and cancer.

It appears we may have ruined our health on the way to the top, because of the lack of care and attention. Don't beat yourself up about it. The real negative factor was just not knowing. Nobody in their right mind would deliberately shorten their life.

But through the folly of doctors and personal doubt or confusion about the issues, we chose to ignore good advice. It's rather like ignoring a good investment and then in later life wishing we had bought shares in something important, for which the value has continuously gone up over the years.

Preserve Your Health Coupons
While on the metaphor of value and investments, let me say this: **You have to look after your health coupons!**

The truth is, health and vitality is a choice. While many may think health is dished out to us at random, it's not so. Health has to be earned. It works like an investment - a little set aside each week or month will result in fruitful rewards in later years. Sadly, far too many individuals squander their health resources and discover all too late that by a certain age their bank account is empty, and all the credits used up. Zip – Nada – Zilch!

We have a state welfare scheme but unfortunately, the government doesn't issue health coupons. You have a full set when you are born (usually) and it is up to you to store these carefully and, if possible, get a return on the investment!

The fact is, for the majority of us alive today, you can say we won't live longer unless we are healthier. Adding years to your life is also a matter of adding life to your years! The few old crocks are the exception by far the majority of men and women who have lived beyond 90 are exceptionally spry and clear-headed for their age.

Do not fear aging. Fear disease but be elated that it is preventable.

So where is all this leading?
As the average Western life expectancy steadily increases, more and more people are going to live beyond the age they imagined they would. Since you will probably to be one of them, it's important you don't find yourself reaching later years with your health a broken property. All it takes is a little intelligent care now, to reap the advantages later.

Get rid of the bravura that "I don't care, I'll take what's coming," because you cannot possibly know how you will feel about this in later years. You might meet someone wonderful or start a new direction in life that would fulfill all your wildest dreams, yet your delight ends up cut short because you haven't taken care of yourself properly.

I have already quoted the American Academy of Anti-Aging Medicine's standpoint: that 50% of Boomers now in good health will live to be over 100. If you found yourself one of the lucky ones, wouldn't it be great if you could enjoy life, even then? But you would want each day to be an experience to look forward to, not to wake up thinking "Oh God, another awful day to get through!" or something equally negative.

The fact is, you may not be able to choose when you die. It would be a tragedy to have to endure a forlorn aching old age, with your body ruined, yet be unable to depart this life quietly and so have to continue to suffer it. Even if euthanasia ever became law (unlikely) it would never be available to those who have simply made a mess of things and lost their enjoyment of life, due to creaking joints, fading hearing and eyesight, physical weakness and general decrepitude.

Actually, it all boils down to being intelligent. Only a fool would squander his or her future in the silly belief that nothing else exciting could happen in life. We already hear about the "Third Age" in life (retirement and beyond); those who have reached it in good shape are finding immense pleasures in life, travelling, finding new hobbies, meeting new friends and, yes, let's not be coy having a vigorous and fulfilling sex life long after the menopause or the male equivalent we've nick-named the "andropause".

> At the age of 75, you still have 85% of the brain cells you were born with

Science To The Rescue

The good news is you can control the outcome. There's plenty of science to guide you down the right path, and I'll help you become clear on the facts.

A keynote study published in the New England Journal of Medicine in 1990 actually showed that aging can be reversed by 10-15 years, as judged by loss of skin wrinkles, increased strength, and muscle mass, reduction in obesity and, of course, feeling great. Even now two decades later, that's totally in disagreement with the word being spread by the average medical practitioner. It's like the medical profession doesn't want an answer to aging!

Intravenous antioxidant therapy, now widely used around the world, can actually reverse the degeneration of arteries and beat free radical damage, so that more oxygen is supplied to important tissues, such as the kidneys, which excrete toxins, and of course the brain.

Here is a unique and safe substance, which appears to re-open arterial pathways and gets more oxygen to the tissues. Some people are finding they no longer require heart by-pass surgery, and blood pressure, as well as angina improves, without the use of drugs. The benefits quickly become available.

In my practice, I pioneered using an entirely new and brilliant additive to these infusions, demonstrated by US doctors providing outstanding benefits to brain functions. People with neurological conditions like Alzheimer's and other dementias, Parkinsonism, stroke, and Multiple Sclerosis had remarkable symptom turn-around. I believe everyone should experience these benefits and move back their date with old age.

Of course there is controversy, but coming from individuals who refuse to objectively acknowledge recent scientific studies' progress. "I didn't think of it, therefore it's bunk", seems to be an all-too-pervasive attitude in medical science these days, with everyone jostling for research grants and prize nominations.

#3. Destructive vs. Constructive Metabolism

My colleague Stephen Cherniske (who incidentally, almost started the anti-aging revolution, with the publication of his book *"DHEA Breakthrough"*) has written about what he called the "Metabolic Breakthrough."

He explains there is a metabolic model of aging. Scientifically, they divide metabolism into 2 main functions (modes): **anabolism**, or building up body and tissues; and **catabolism**, the breaking down of body and tissues. Anabolism is the building and repair process; catabolism is the clearing away of decay and waste products.

As children, we are almost entirely in anabolic mode, as we need to continue to build and grow vigorously. But from the age of 20- 25, this process stops. This is when we are at our peak, and that's about as good as our health gets! From there on, it's all downhill, known as the catabolism stage.

In health, these two must remain in reasonable balance. But as we age, gradually catabolism (the processes of decay) takes over more and more. The faster it goes, the quicker we age.

Cherniske uses the model of a seesaw: on one side we have the forces of repair and regeneration, on the other side, the forces of damage and decay. Kids sit comfortably on the up side of the seesaw and seem to repair with astonishing speed, even when they become seriously sick or injured. Inevitably, our rejuvenation ration gets used up, as we get older. The seesaw starts to go down on our side! The trick is to hold back the decay part and hang on to the repair and regeneration mode for as long as you can.

When you reach the age of 50, if you accept the generous estimate of A4M (page 7) your life is about half over. The trouble is, it's the fun half that went before. As we get older, the steady erosion gradually leads us towards disease, decline, and decrepitude. Certainly not something we want to accept without a fight.

It's important for you to grasp this bitter truth, because if you just treat aging as a cosmetic affair and try to paper over the cracks, you'll die on your allotted day! If you want to survive the longest possible time with the maximum attainable level of vigor, you must address the forces of decay and disintegration. Until you learn to hold them in check, you will simply continue to go down until you inevitably die.

We can now test our anabolic vs. catabolic status with an ingenious test. It's called the ACI (anabolic/catabolic index) and it measures critical anabolic metabolites, called 17 ketosteroid sulfates (or sulphates for the Europeans). These 17-KS-S levels rise when the body goes into determined heal and repair mode. They are diminished or lacking in catabolic states.

The sample required is urine and then you can tell quickly and conveniently exactly how fast you are aging. Stephen Cherniske carried out a trial showing that nutritional intervention can restore ACI levels, so neatly closing the circle.

The manual you are now holding is filled with great ideas of ways you can drive your ACI back into the health zone. Make the most of it! It's exciting that suddenly at your fingertips is the kind of help you need to not just live longer but live longer with good health.

#4. A Note on Dying

Woody Allen once said, "I don't mind dying. I just don't want to be there when it happens." And while I like what he has to say, the fact of the matter is we cannot avoid the topic of death.

The real Japanese Samurai warriors (from before the 20th century) had a fetish about dying a "good death". While it may sound like an oxymoron, these warriors would rather die in a blaze of glory than go on to an ignominious old age and just fade away.

> **Medical science is crude, simplistic, biased, ignorant, narrow-minded, and dangerous.**

Thing is, it's not one or the other. There is a "third way", to use Buddha's term.

It makes sense to live a long and glorious life and enjoy it right to the last day. Sooner or later, it all must come to an end. But to me the really important part of anti-aging is living life to the fullest while we are here. How long we spend on planet Earth is less important as long as we truly "live." So it's time to start being prudent with the health coupons we were issued with as a baby!

Avoiding the Speed Bumps!

The Center for Disease Control reported the top 10 causes of death for 2005 were as follows:
1. Heart disease
2. Cancer
3. Stroke
4. Chronic lower respiratory diseases (lung diseases)
5. Accidents
6. Diabetes
7. Alzheimer's disease

8. Influenza and pneumonia
9. Kidney disease
10. Septicemia (a serious infection that affects the blood)

These were closely followed by suicide, chronic liver disease and cirrhosis, high blood pressure, Parkinson's disease and homicide.

The CDC also reports the top three causes of death -- heart disease, cancer, and stroke -- declined in 2005, compared with 2004, leading to greater life expectancy. However, heart disease, cancer, and stroke remain the country's top killers. The life expectancy statistics are based on the CDC's preliminary data on more than 2.4 million deaths nationwide in 2005.

Statistics Can Lie

Don't get bogged down with statistics. What's really important is what happens to YOU, not what happens to others. You're not a statistic, you're not even average. We are all different. I only want you to understand that the old-fashioned idea of a generation ago was you were pretty well finished by your 70s, and there was nothing much you could do about it. This is **false** and has always been false.

If you go to other societies considered less fortunate, you'll find living beyond 100 has always been pretty common. I first noticed this among my Scottish ancestors, living to 90-100 years, on a diet of herring and oatmeal (there are good reasons why these would help you live long). They also had plenty of exercise, walked long distances and, by the way, drank plenty of whisky.

So my first piece of advice for living healthy and long is *ignore everything you are told by regular doctors!* I mean it! Medical science is crude, simplistic, biased, ignorant, narrow-minded, and dangerous. Most of it is, after all, centered around drug company profits, not patient care in the true sense of the word.

You need renegade doctors that can think outside the box. Yes, I'm putting myself forward. I can't think of anyone better qualified to do it!

How Many Bumps Did You Say?

But wait—didn't I say there were just 6 main speed bumps in the road? Yes, that's right.

Many of these figures are quite complicated and don't necessarily speak the truth. For example, someone paralyzed by a stroke but survives, only to die in bed of pneumonia (a very common outcome), would not show up as a stroke death in the statistics. But really a stroke was the cause of the fatality; pneumonia and respiratory disease is thus exaggerated. In any case, 4 and 8 on the CDC list are pretty similar.

Stroke and heart disease are also pretty much the same thing, under different names. Whether the heart is most affected or the brain, the actual disease is arteriosclerosis or bad arteries. Even Alzheimer's can be seen as a disease of the circulatory system, since the main problem seems to be poor nutrient blood supply to the brain, caused by aging arteries.

We can rule out accidents, since avoiding them is hardly a medical matter. To die in a car crash has nothing to do with the aging process! It's just tough luck.

So! We can actually boil the top of the list down to this:

1. Aging circulation
2. Cancer
3. Diabetes
4. Kidney disease
5. Septicemia.

But that's only 5 what about the 6th speed bump in the road to death?

This is what they didn't tell you in the report: **doctors are the 3rd leading cause of death in the US!** These account for over 225,000 deaths per year [Journal American Medical Association 2000 Jul 26;284(4):483-5]*. "Iatrogenic" causes, they are called, a Greek word, which means, "caused by doctors".

Doctors Are the Number One Killers

*According to Dr Barbara Starfield, who prepared the report for The Journal of the American Medical Association (JAMA is the largest and one of the most respected medical journals in the entire world), doctors are actually the number one killer, because they do not inform patients properly of the hazards of the procedures they offer. Then again, why would they? The patient might have second thoughts and that would mean lost income for the doctor!

Therefore, my first piece of critical advice is if you want to live a long and healthy life, you need to stay away from doctors and hospitals. They are by far the biggest speed bump in your way. In fact, when doctors go on strike ironically the death rate always drops.

It is an incredible irony that when the doctors in Colombia went on strike, the death rate plummeted by thirty-five percent, only to resume its "normal" level when work resumed. When doctors in Los Angeles went on a work slow-down in 1976 to protest soaring malpractice insurance premiums, the death rate dropped by eighteen percent. Again in Israel in 1973 when the doctors reduced their daily patient contact from 65,000 to 7,000, during a month long strike, the death rate dropped fifty percent during that month, according to the Jerusalem Burial Society. (Mendelsohn R. Confessions Of A Medical Heretic, Contemporary Books, Chicago, 1979, p. 114)

So I will guide you through the minefield of lies and disinformation that abounds in health care. Some of it comes from ignorant doctors and scientists but plenty comes from alternative "health practitioners," many of who are on the make and speak falsely to make dollars. Believe me!

Cancer and Heart Disease

Between 80 and 90% of deaths are directly related to heart disease and cancer. Yet the formula for beating these conditions is the same, really, as preventing aging. The benefit to you, as a committed anti-ager, is that you dramatically improve your chances against these two diseases. It comes as a bonus!

The truth is, over and over again, it has been demonstrated these are preventable conditions. Don't be fooled by the trigger factors, such as tobacco smoking and lung cancer. Not everyone who smokes gets cancer and not everyone who gets lung cancer has smoked; the late Roy Castle was a famous example of this. He got lung cancer yet had never smoked in his life. Therefore, there are other factors at work.

These other factors include nutrition, moderate lifestyle, a cleaner environment, and personal health care. Similarly, the "genes-for-everything" scientists, who keep announcing that everything from cancer to homosexuality is just a gene are being very unscientific. It will help you appreciate this if you realize there is huge money in genetics. What you are hearing is the voice of greed, not the voice of science.

Most of these announcements turn out to be completely false. While this sort of propagandizing does the price of stockholders shares a lot of good, it does nothing for human health! Almost all known causes of cancer and heart disease are environmental, meaning outside the body. You can control them! Children who "inherit" from their parents also inherit bad diet and lifestyle factors, don't forget this important fact. It doesn't take the heroic effort of a monastic lifestyle.

There is another misconception to work round. There is a widely held belief that being healthy means behaving like a freak and missing out on all the fun. This is just not true. It's an attitude of being childish and indulgent for a few years and then advancing into chronic and not very pleasant health conditions.

The same mentality would allow a family or tribe to starve, because it was too much trouble to plant next year's crops and water the seedlings. Until the twentieth century that would have literally cost you your life. It's the same sensible husbandry with your health. Take a little care now, think ahead, and you can reap the harvest of goodness for many years to come.

1 | What Exactly Is Aging? Anti-Aging Models

We have still to learn exactly what aging is. We can observe it happening but that doesn't mean we understand it. In fact, some animals don't seem to age at all, while others like the tortoise age very, very slowly. That only makes matters all the more mysterious. However, medical science is now showing an intense interest in aging, and a huge amount of money is now being spent on researching aging mechanisms and how to prevent them (because there is big money potential in it, of course, not because they care!)

A number of key mechanisms of aging have been suggested, some of which need to be considered.

Oxidative Damage Model

Probably the most widely accepted view of aging is that it is steady tissue degeneration, caused by oxidative damage – exactly like the rusting of iron. It is interesting to note that oxygen – so necessary for life – is also a serious poison. Just a few percentage increases in oxygen levels, over a few hours, causes blindness and then cell death. Oxygen brings life but the great irony is that every breath we take we die a little.

Biologists believe that probably the only reason we have evolved life on earth is because of the coincident development of antioxidant mechanisms within cells, especially the mitochondria. You will hear, time and time again, that survival comes back to antioxidant mechanisms. What does that mean?

Oxygen itself is not so bad but in certain enhanced forms, it is a deadly destroyer. We call these "reactive oxygen species" (ROS) and they interact violently with almost all chemical compounds, changing and damaging them. That includes substances within our bodies, particularly the precious cell membranes, which are mostly lipids (fatty) and so turn rancid at the least whiff of oxygen.

Reactive oxygen is only one of a whole family of substances called "free radicals". They are not exactly free but they are sure damned hungry. They munch at anything nearby and anything bitten in turn becomes a new reactive molecule, so it goes on the hunger prowl, and so. It's a self-perpetuating chain and bad news for immortalists (those who want to live forever).

Other free radicals include reactive nitrogen species (RNS), hydroxyl radicals (the –OH of chemistry), peroxide (which is so deadly our white cells use it in a controlled way to kill microbes prior to eating them) and, quite a surprise, iron which in its free radical form I have christened "hot iron" and is probably the most deadly of all.

If you are wondering why it is that Nature seems to have gotten it all wrong, you are not alone.

Fortunately, provided we have an adequate supply of antioxidants in the body, we get along, as life has been doing nicely for over half a billion years! You will hear of the "master guardian" superoxidase dismutase (SOD), which is the anti-oxygen vigilante and two others, equally important: catalase, which destroys peroxide, and glutathione reducatase which attacks the hydroxyl ion.

But many other substances can act as antioxidants, that is *oxygen killers*, simply by satisfying that horrible hunger of the free radicals. Vitamin C, vitamin E, beta-carotenoids, and selenium were among the first to be recognized.

One of the most powerful, second only to SOD, is glutathione and its precursors N-acetyl cysteine, and alpha lipoic acid. Now we know there are scores, from flavonoids in red wine, polyphenols in chocolate, catechins in tea, quercetin in onions (cooked or raw), anthocyanins in blue-black fruits, and the "sleep" hormone melatonin, to name just a few.

We are now certain that free radical damage is a crucial mechanism of aging, even if it is not the only one, so you must take steps to safeguard yourself.

See Chapter 8 for more advice on antioxidants.

Genes Model

A common question about aging is whether or not genes have an important role to play. In other words, does it matter who your ancestors are and does that have much bearing on how long you will live?

Today it's fashionable to believe that everything is in the genes. But genes don't always show up. The gene for blue eyes, for instance, is subordinate to the gene for brown eyes. So if you get one of each (one from your mother and one from your father), the brown eyes will win. This is called a *dominant gene* (blue eyes are a *recessive gene*).

But then it is found that sometimes even the dominant gene doesn't show up, as it should. So scientists began to talk of gene "expression" (whether it will come into play or not).

Many external factors will influence whether or not a gene expresses itself fully or partially. We call these factors *epi-genetics* (*epi-* means stuck on top, like skin or epidermis). Without question, the number one epigenetic factor is diet and nutrition. It has been demonstrated, over and over, that changing what you eat will change the expression of dangerous genes.

Really all this is saying that environmental factors are very important and genes are not the be-all-and-end-all, though science continues to peddle this silly story as if genes were absolute in their force.

Where does this leave us in anti-aging science? There are many genetic factors that are being studied right now. One is in relation to calorie-restricted diets. Dr, Stephen R. Spindler, Professor at the Department of Biochemistry at the University of California, Riverside, has studied the effect of long- and short-term CR diets on the expression of some 11,000 age-related genes in animals. He found something remarkable and published it in the Proceedings of the National Academy of Sciences (September 11, 2001).

Not only was the age-benefit effect of CR seen over and over again but genetically determined age changes could be **reversed**. Till then, science had assumed that the genes took effect but the resulting damaging changes were blocked by CR. What Spindler showed, using sophisticated microchip technology, was that the expression of many pro-aging genes was actually reversed.

The good news was that this occurred even in elderly animals. Because the effect was not merely blocking damage but undoing gene expression, they became younger animals, so to speak. Naturally, some genes decrease their expression due to aging; Spindler found.

It is interesting that Spindler found that 40% of the genes that increased expression with age were associated with inflammatory changes and 25% associated with oxidative stress. You will learn through this report that inflammation is one of the key processes of aging; according to this finding, it's more critical than the oxidative damage that is supposed to head the list of aging causes.

No wonder food restriction helps survival, if it reduces inflammation and other stresses. It would also explain the benefits of Luigi Cornaro's diet (**page 58**) and indeed any detox plan.

HOT TIP

I can't recommend full CR dieting for humans; the levels used in the animal experiments were very drastic. But you could consider three immediate actions:

- Reduce your calorie intake significantly, even if not to the point of hunger, starting right NOW
- Consider a 1, 2 or 3-day fast as a substitute for CR dieting
- A weekly one-day grape/juice or full fast. That's 52 days a year of knocking back gene expression!

Look out for drugs that will mimic CR diets. None are yet on the market but there is a race to get them to you.

To learn more about genes and aging and the work of Dr Stephen R. Spindler, visit www.lifespangenetics.com. His work has been funded by the Life Extension Foundation: www.lef.org

Carbohydrate Control Model (Insulin Resistance)

One of the absolute benchmarks for longevity is keeping carbs under control. Specifically, having a lower blood insulin than average. It seems there's a great deal of research that indicates that lower the carbs, and you'll not only increase your longevity, you'll increase the quality of your health.

> **The current obesity epidemic is one of the toughest health challenges faced today.**

The current obesity epidemic is one of the toughest health challenges faced today. Fat and carbohydrate consumption have been directly linked to poor health, while protein is largely ignored. Yet protein has been the constant in civilizations where longevity and health go hand in hand.

You'll learn about the so-called metabolic syndrome, which is still being researched and gradually understood in the aging context. It seems that carbohydrates are very powerful in their damaging effect on our bodies. Even whole grains and complex carbohydrates are not that safe. Remember, grains are farmer foods and not natural to a hunter-gatherer creature, such as we are in evolutionary terms.

Telomeres and DNA Damage Model

Another important model of aging is the progressive denaturing of our DNA, the genetic messenger. DNA regulates most or all of the metabolic processes which go on in our cells. If the DNA messages become damaged, or corrupted, then the cells may begin to behave weirdly. Telomeres are strands on the ends of our chromosomes that are supposed to prevent this decay process.

Telomeres consist of up to 3,300 repeats of the DNA sequence TTAGGG. They protect chromosome ends from being mistaken for broken pieces of DNA that would otherwise be fixed by cellular repair machinery. But every time our cells divide, the telomeres shrink. When they get short enough, our cells no longer divide and our body stops making those cells. Over time, this leads to aging and death. Babies have lots of an enzyme called *telomerase*, which repairs the telomeres, but we lose that steadily through time as well. It seems to be inactive in normal adult cells.

Certainly one of the reasons cancer is seen increasingly as age advances is that telomere loss makes it more and more likely to occur. Interestingly, cancer cells have high levels of telomerase enzyme and so can continue to repair their telomeres, which is why they go on vigorously growing and dividing.

There is no question that the telomere mechanism is crucial to aging, though many would not accept that this is the cause of aging so much as a *result* of aging processes, such as oxidative damage, which certainly decreases the telomere count.

Still, it's pretty clear telomeres are significant. One study of centenarians showed they had significantly longer telomeres than average [Delara et al. "Association of Longer Telomeres With Better Health in Centenarians." The Journals of Gerontology Series A: Biological Sciences and Medical Sciences. 208. 63:809-812.]

Hot Off the Press

A few aging cells isn't much of a problem. But a startling new July 2010 study now shows that people who accumulate a lot of cells with short telomeres have a greatly increased risk of fatal cancers.

Compared to people at the top third of average telomere length, those at the bottom third have a threefold higher risk of cancer. Those in the middle third have twice the cancer risk as those with the longest telomeres.

"Of note, telomere length was preferentially associated with individual cancers characterized by a high fatality rate such as gastric, lung, and ovarian cancer -- but less so with tumors linked to better prognosis," found Peter Willeit, MD, of Austria's Innsbruck Medical University, and colleagues.

Those in the lowest third of telomere length were over 11 times more likely to die of cancer than those in the highest third. Those in the middle third were 5.6 times more likely to die of cancer.

For 10 years, Willeit's team followed 787 residents of Bruneck, Italy, who received all their medical care at the same local hospital. Ranging in age from 40 to 79, all were cancer free at the beginning of the study. A decade later, 92 of the study participants had developed cancer.

At regular intervals, the researchers calculated the average telomere length of each participant's white blood cells. This led to a number of interesting findings:

Men had shorter telomeres than women.
Short telomere length was linked to risk of diabetes and chronic infection.
Short telomere length was linked to increased risk of several killer cancers.
Short telomere length was not linked to breast or colon cancer.
Short telomere length was associated with lack of physical exercise.

[Willeit, P. Journal of the American Medical Association, July 7, 2010; vol 304: pp 69-75]

HOT TIP

You can get a telomerase count, an enzyme which tells you how you are doing and whether you have active cancer or not (cancer cells have 10-20 the levels of telomerase of ordinary cells). Originally, a urine test, it is now available reliably as a blood test. A relatively high telomerase count is indicative of active cancer in the body. This test may soon be adopted as a means of screening high-risk patients and detecting tumors long before they grow to significant size.

Help Your Telomeres

You can boost your telomeres by up to 30% (29%), according to an article published in the *Lancet* journal in 2008, by the means of judicious lifestyle changes. The program used in the study was as follows:

A low-fat (10% of calories from fat), whole foods, plant-based diet high in fruits, vegetables, unrefined grains, legumes, and low in refined carbohydrates; moderate aerobic exercise (walking 30 min/day, 6 days/week); stress management (gentle yoga-based stretching, breathing, meditation, imagery, and progressive relaxation techniques 60 min/day, 6 days/week), and a 1h group support session once per week.

The diet was supplemented with soy (one daily serving of tofu plus 58 g of a fortified soy protein powdered beverage), fish oil (3 g daily), vitamin E (100 IU daily), selenium (200 µg daily), and vitamin C (2 g daily). [Ornish et al. "Increased telomerase activity and comprehensive lifestyle changes: a pilot study." The Lancet Oncology. 2008. 9(11):1048-1057].

I think the important take-away here is not what the lifestyle changes were, exactly, but that if you care to make sensible changes, you will benefit from it in increased longevity. That's what this entire book is about!

Stress Model

Everyone (I think) knows that stress is a killer. We'll deal with that more later when we come to ask why the Pacific salmon ages and dies so dramatically after spawning and how this is relevant to human aging. It is important to have this model in your mind, when you are considering different modes of biological aging processes.

Remember stress is not just bankruptcy, divorce, or being made redundant. Lack of sleep is stress (important too); a viral infection is stress; chemical exposure is stress; having dental transplants or fillings is stress; economic crisis is stress; global warming is stress… and so on.

Stress is activated primarily through hormones, particularly the so-called HPA (hypophyseal-pituitary-adrenal pathways) axis.

Killer Cortisol

Today we understand the biological basis of stress far better than just a few decades ago. Formerly stress was viewed simply in terms of adrenalin rush and the short-range dangers of stress when continued long term. Adrenalin (epinephrine) is the "flight or fight" hormone, which gears up the body for sudden exertion in times of danger.

Unfortunately, today, we live lives of almost constant stress. When stress becomes chronic, a different mechanism kicks in; one which is dangerous and ultimately exhausting. It literally drains the life from your body. You don't want that.

I'm talking about the hormone cortisol. It too comes from the adrenal gland but a different part from adrenalin. Let me tell you how dangerous cortisol is, by resorting to some biology; I'll talk about the life and death of the Pacific salmon.

I'm sure you know the story: salmon come in from the ocean to reproduce; they migrate up river; they mate and spawn and then, their purpose fulfilled, they die dramatically. Hundreds of thousands of diseased fish corpses are washed back towards the sea.

The journey upriver is dramatic and stressful; the fish have to get up huge waterfalls and cataracts; they don't eat and struggle continuously for days. That's stress!

As a result, their cortisol levels rise by over a thousand-fold and that's what kills them. In just a few days after spawning, the lethal levels of cortisol wipe out the salmon's immune system; many become infected with pathogens. They die quickly, as a direct result of raised cortisol.

This is a fishy example, but cortisol is just as bad for us. We don't get elevations of a thousand-fold. But even moderately raised cortisol levels are dangerous. You need to keep it under control.

High cortisol levels are associated with a number of premature aging mechanisms: impaired immune system, loss of fertility, diminished bone strength, abdominal weight gain, loss of verbal declarative memory, insulin resistance, and Type 2 Diabetes Mellitus, to name just a few.

You need to avoid stress as much as possible, if you want a long and healthy life. Period!

Inflammation Model

The final model of aging we want to discuss here is that of inflammation. It's quite simply the number one cause of aging, period!

Many degenerative diseases of aging have an inflammatory basis and on closer examination, this emerges as a very significant factor in telling us why the body deteriorates rapidly in some individuals and much more slowly in others. What's more, it is something we can test for quite easily and thereby gain the advantage of a health marker that tells us exactly how we are progressing.

Degenerative Inflammatory Diseases

The following are just some of the many degenerative diseases in humans, which have an inflammatory nature:

- Arteriosclerosis
- Alzheimer's disease
- Parkinson's disease
- Lupus
- Asthma
- Kidney failure
- Diabetes
- Pancreatitis
- Arthritis (especially rheumatoid)
- Allergy
- ME or fibromyalgia
- Cancer
- Liver failure and cirrhosis
- Multiple sclerosis

Sources of Inflammation

One of the newest sources of chronic inflammation to be recognized comes from what we call "stealth pathogens". These are invasive organisms: viruses, bacteria and even parasites, which keep a low profile and do not set off a very overt disease process and so they pass unnoticed, often without raising the wrath of the immune system.

Organisms known to behave in this way are *Chlamydia pneumoniae*, certain herpes viruses (shingles, for example, is the chicken pox herpes virus, which has lain hidden and dormant for decades before erupting), cytomegalovirus, Epstein-Barr. Many people suffering from ME are harboring an unknown stealth pathogen. Certainly, *Candida albicans* may be one of these but probably not as often as is claimed. There may even be *nanobacteria*, so tiny they have never been seen until recent years, which some investigators are convinced underlie a lot of health problems. I'm not convinced about nanobacteria.

Remember, not all inflammatory origins are infective in nature. A great deal of it comes from what we call auto-immune diseases: disorders in which the body attacks itself, using inappropriate antibodies. Rheumatoid arthritis, lupus, Hashimoto's thyroiditis and a great many other diseases have a strong auto-immune component.

Severe exertion also generates an inflammatory process within the body, releasing many white cells, and increasing the marker substances discussed below. Physical activity is vital against aging but excessive effort is certainly counter-productive.

Once again, this may explain a paradox: why people who spend so much time in the gym do not always survive longer. Working out too much can damage your health – exactly as Dr Li Ching-Yun stated!

Inflammation can also be chemical-based. Pollutants that settle in belly fat have been found to be particularly damaging because of the inflammation pathways they excite (see next section). Most notorious are the excito-toxins, dangerous food additives, and heavy metal poisons, such as lead mercury and aluminum. We deal with these in a separate section (page 210).

Vaccinations may also play a part and linger in a destructive way. I am convinced, through over 40 years of clinical work and research, that vaccinations upset the immune system and that this can lead to auto-immune attacks on our own tissues. However, medical science is simply not ready for this admission yet, though many other doctors report seeing it daily in their practice and know it is happening.

Finally, unresolved illnesses may go underground, only to emerge later as chronic degenerative disease. Holistic doctors have been arguing for years that treatments with many modern drugs have simply driven the disease process out of view, and that the process continues unresolved, even when symptoms are effectively masked.

At present, these views are regarded as mere hearsay within the medical profession. But you have two expert opinions here pointing out the concern. There is no need to wait for hesitant medical science to catch up, if the warning signs are clear. Remember the food industry and drug cartels do not want you to learn the truth about their products. They control the medical schools and pay for most of the scientific research in universities.

The Hayflick Limit

I cannot leave the topic of aging models without reference to this giant red herring. It crops up all the time.

In 1965, Leonard Hayflick published a paper in which he claimed to have proved that cells artificially kept in a test tube environment can only divide about 50 times and then they die. This would imply that potential human life span was limited and nothing could be done, because once the 50 divisions were used up, the person was doomed. In keeping with science tradition, this discovery is known as the "Hayflick Limit". Mainstream science has grabbed at this gloomy prediction and acts as if it were a proven case. It is not.

One reason to think Hayflick was wrong is that every cell now in existence is a daughter cell of an earlier cell and an earlier, earlier and so on, right back to the dawn of life! Put that way, at best Hayflick showed there may be some change in cell activity at the point of fusion of the sperm and egg (conception), which effectively puts the clock back to zero.

Some of us think all Hayflick really proved was he didn't know much about cell nutrition and physiology! Some cancer cells are tough hardy brutes and go on indefinitely, thousands of times beyond the Hayflick limit. There is no logical reason, other than our ignorance of their detailed requirements, that ordinary cells cannot do the same, if they are given the right milieu.

Interestingly, more recent science has shown that normal cells within the body survive longer than those in a test tube. Also certain bone marrow cells have been shown to escape the Hayflick Limit, and so the whole question is still very open.

The really important point is that we could all live a long, long time, *within the Hayflick limit*, if only we reduce the rate of cell damage and thus cell replacement. Experts have calculated that even if the Hayflick limit were true, the number of permissible cell divisions would equate to a human life span of 300 years. That's an average, so many of us could live far longer, if we wished!

Maybe there was a Methuselah?

Attitude is Crucial

There's an old saying, "You are as old as you feel." No question: how you view yourself and your state of health affects not just how long you will live but the quality of your life.

We all know it; but yet another study proved it.

Researchers found older people with positive views on aging were 44% more likely to recover fully after severe disability than those with negative views on aging.

In the study, researchers periodically surveyed 598 people aged 70 or older about their views on aging over a period of about 11 years.

None were disabled when the study started, but later on, all of them had at least one month when they needed help with daily tasks such as bathing, dressing, or walking. In some cases, their disability was severe; other cases were mild.

They were asked for the first five words or phrases that come to mind when they think of old people. The researchers rated their responses on a five-point scale as most positive, like "spry," or most negative, like "decrepit."

Quite simply, those who viewed aging with horror and put themselves in the old age category had a poorer outlook on life, worse health and did not live as long.

The results appeared in the Nov. 21, 2012, Journal of the American Medical Association.

2 | Emotional Longevity

Here's where we truly go "outside the box". There are certain factors that appear crucial to aging healthily and attaining a degree of longevity. Yet most writers ignore these and plough on solely about vitamins, anti-oxidants, insulin levels, exercise, etc, as if these more mind-based aspects of our make-up didn't count.

Aging, as we shall see in this section, is not just about biology. Mind and spirit too are critical. Hardly surprising, since we now know the importance of the mind-body connection.

Emotional longevity is a term coined by Norman B. Anderson, Ph.D., the CEO of the American Psychological Association, and the author of the book titled, *Emotional Longevity: What Really Determines How Long You Live*. A former professor at both Duke University Medical School and Harvard School of Public Health, Anderson also is the former and founding associate director of the National Institutes of Health (NIH) in charge of behavioral and social sciences research.

Anderson looked way outside the usual box, into behaviors and society - genetics, environmental pressures, social networks, and marital status. What really determines how long you live and how happy you are with your life?

Emotional longevity, says Anderson, is about connections — connections between biology and social relationships; among biology, beliefs, and behavior; and between biology and emotions. We have long believed some of these connections are important, and science has now confirmed them as such, but other connections are much more surprising.

Research that tracks large groups of healthy people throughout several years finds that a certain percentage of these people died prematurely from illnesses that were not predicted based on their age, initial health, or established risk factors such as poor diet, lack of exercise, biological risk, or family medical history. Clearly, something is missing from our ability to predict longevity, and Anderson suggests a need to broaden our definition of health and its determinants.

Why do some people with seemingly the same health profile enjoy good physical health while others become sick? And why among patients with the same illnesses do some recover while others do not? In the last few decades, science has been inching closer to providing answers. In fact, a large volume of health research now points to a new definition of health that is multifaceted and includes the previously missing pieces.

A number of these pieces are surprising and not obviously physiological at all. In his fascinating book, Anderson has assembled an impressive array of scientifically sound research identifying five additional dimensions as key determinants of health and longevity, other than biology:

- Thoughts and actions
- Environment and relationships
- Personal achievement and equality
- Emotions and stress
- Faith and meaning

What may be new to you is the way each of these factors is strongly and unequivocally connected to physical illness and longevity. Moreover, as Anderson emphasizes, all these factors are strongly interconnected and capable of influencing each other, for better or for worse. Let's look at each in turn.

Thoughts and Actions

The importance of actions (e.g., "lifestyle" factors) to health is well known. But what is less recognized is the importance of thought processes and the fact that how we view the world can also be predictive of health outcomes. For example, optimists, who tend to expect more positive outcomes and interpret the past in ways that are more uplifting, have been found to live longer, recover faster from surgery, have lower mortality from cancer, and fewer chronic illnesses than pessimists.

Another example is the fact that people who write deeply and thoughtfully about traumatic experiences have fewer health problems than those who do not. Research by psychologist James Pennebaker Ph.D. and others finds that disclosure through writing or other means can improve mood, decrease doctor visits, boost the immune system, and improve perceived health.

To see if this technique works for you, Pennebaker recommends that you pick a topic that you think needs some resolution and then set aside 15 minutes to write continuously over several days. It doesn't have to be an extremely stressful or traumatic event — just something important to you that is perhaps difficult to express to others.

If you are a talker more than a writer, try talking into a tape recorder, which research indicates produces comparable results to writing. Either way, try to explore your deepest thoughts and feelings. Describe what happened, how you feel about it, and why you might feel that way. You may have more feelings that are negative immediately after writing, but usually these do not last very long. In time, your emotional well-being should improve.

Environment and Relationships

Having a supportive social network is predictive of lower mortality, faster recovery from heart attacks, fewer common colds, slower progression to AIDS in HIV-positive patients, and less atherosclerosis in the coronary arteries.

One of the strongest contexts for getting and receiving social support is marriage. More than 100 years of research finds that a good marriage is good for your health. Married people live longer and have fewer chronic diseases than do single, widowed, or divorced people. While married people have a higher socioeconomic position on average (a protective factor in itself) than people who are not married, the influence of social support seems to be a key reason that married people live longer.

> **Married people live longer and have fewer chronic diseases than do single, widowed, or divorced people.**

It's notable also that those who have been married and are now divorced enjoy better health and less senility than those who never married but not as good as those who remain happily married. There does seem to be some scientific truth then in the old adage from the poet Tennyson: "Tis better to have loved and lost than never to have loved at all"!

Personal Achievement and Equality

Statistics show that people who have lower levels of educational attainment, income, and occupational status, which together have been labeled "socioeconomic status" are at greater risk for early mortality than people higher on these scales. In addition, the greater the distance between the rich and the poor, in a country or a state, the greater the annual mortality in the entire population.

Why? In addition to influencing our exposure to chronic stress, socioeconomic status plays a huge, perhaps dominant, role in the options available to us and the decisions we make. Choice, flexibility, and control over life's important aspects vary with socioeconomic status. The more options you have, the more flexibility you have about how you spend your time, and the greater your sense of control over your life in general.

This sense of control and empowerment may be especially important for health, since research suggests that not having them can be deadly. The effects of not having control are striking in the work setting. People in very demanding or physically taxing jobs with little control are at higher risk for heart disease and mortality. Recent research indicates that the truly toxic element of work strain is not high demand; rather, a low level of job control is a deadly ingredient.

As well as status, when researched the sense of personal achievement proved important. I don't know if you saw the movie "About Schmidt", starring Jack Nicholson (based on the book by Louis Begley). Schmidt is a man who arrives at retirement age and realizes he has achieved NOTHING. His life has been a patent waste and he is brought face to face with his inadequate self.

Schmidt tries to paper over the gaps by making himself valuable to former colleagues and his daughter but in fact, he becomes an irritating nuisance to them. They reject him. Finally, his wife dies and everything collapses about him.

It's an extremely depressing and defeatist story (not close to the book at all). In fact, it's the kind of movie to make you feel like slashing your wrists! But there is a kind of redemption in the last few seconds of the movie. Go see it. Just take some Kleenex.

On the positive side, what enriches life is the sense of real achievement and personal satisfaction.

Emotions and Stress

Emotions are deadly. In fact, they kill faster than anything else. Emotions can trigger inflammation in the body and we've already discussed how inflammation is hazardous to your longevity. You may have also already heard about the relationship between emotion and cortisol levels in the body. Cortisol has been proven to be directly tied to emotions, weight gain, inflammation in the body, and poor health.

We can measure cortisol. Somebody somewhere has probably done the math: so many mgms of cortisol in your blood equals so many years off your life. Some people love to do those sums. I read one decades ago (from America, of course) that every passionate kiss takes 7 minutes off your life. I think it must be flawed science, even if the math is correct, because we now know that love and passion keep us going strong and healthy into our twilight years.

Emotions and Survival

Recent healthcare news has indicated that the effects of negative emotions on the heart can lead to cardiac problems. In fact, research has found that emotional upheaval, whether it is anger, worry, depression, or stress, increases the risk of heart attack and/or stroke.

In 2007, an assistant professor of psychology, at Indiana University, by the name of Jesse Stewart, Ph.D. led a three year research study that was later published in the Archives of General Psychiatry. This research directly linked negative emotions such as the ones previously mentioned, with arthrosclerosis, a condition where the inside wall of the coronary arteries thicken, slowing or blocking the flow of blood.

Dr. Stewart went on to say that this link is not a weak link by any stretch of the imagination. The risk of negative emotions is comparable to any of the other factors pertaining to cardiovascular diseases.

Dr. Stewart says, "Depression can be considered an emerging risk factor for heart disease. It can be thought of as much the same way as cholesterol or high blood pressure or smoking, although the evidence base is not the highest available."

Loneliness

If an empty nest or early retirement leaves you feeling isolated, the heartache may be more than emotional. In a 19-year study, women who reported feeling lonely most of the time had a 76 percent increased risk of heart disease. The connection? Chronic loneliness, like stress, may trigger inflammatory and hormonal changes that promote cardiovascular disease.

It could also be, of course, that people living alone don't look after themselves properly, eating poorly and not taking enough care of personal health issues.

Either way, it makes sense to nurture your friendships and forge close social connections by volunteering at a local charity, joining a book club, or undertaking any other social activities that appeal to you.

The Heart and Negative Emotions

According to clinical psychologist Barry J. Jacobs, Psy.D., a faculty member at the Crozer-Keystone Family Medicine Residency Program in Springfield, Pa., and the American Heart Association spokesperson, there are two main reasons why negative emotions can directly affect the heart.

The first reason has to do with the effects on behavior. If a person is depressed or stressed, it can lead to not taking proper care of oneself and/or participating in activities that are unhealthy. They may drink too much, take recreational drugs, not eat properly, not get proper sleep, or not take medications as prescribed.

Dr. Jacobs says, "There's mounting research that when people get stressed out, their hormonal system produces more cortisol," a hormone released by the adrenal gland. This has been associated with heart disease and diabetes."

Dr. Jacobs also says, "The arteries tend to narrow when people are in situations of very high stress."

The second reason is depression, which can negatively affect the heart. Depression is directly linked to a rise in inflammation in the body, which is measured by markers in the blood. It seems that if these markers are present it can be used to predict a heart attack in the future.

Taking time to take better care of your emotional health can translate to better physical health. A good night's sleep makes it easier to handle stress and makes you less likely to become depressed. Eating a diet rich in whole grains, fruits, and vegetables, while avoiding alcohol and cigarettes is also a great way to reduce the stress in your life, as is yoga, meditation, praying, reading, and just some good old-fashioned quiet time.

We should also mention the importance of music and laughter in keeping the heart healthy. A little fun is great for keeping you overall healthier and younger. It seems laughter really is the best medicine.

With the fun should be a little (or a lot) of relaxation. Relaxation comes in many forms: Meditation, playing a card game with friends, reading, or going for a walk are just a few ways to relax. Relaxation is good for the heart and good for the body, keeping you younger than your years.

Control Over Your Life Status vs. Stress

Contrary to popular supposition, having a highly stressful, demanding job will not necessarily impair your health or shorten your life. What really seems to matter is how much control you have over your work environment.

In fact, leaders and managers enjoy better health and longevity than low-level workers. The reason, when eventually isolated, is the question of having control or being controlled. The latter is highly toxic.

One of the first studies to reach this conclusion was the now-famous "Whitehall Study" conducted among workers in the British civil service (hence Whitehall). The original Whitehall Study investigated social determinants of health, specifically the cardiorespiratory disease prevalence, and mortality rates among British male civil servants between the ages of 20 and 64. The initial study, the Whitehall I Study, was conducted over a period of ten years, beginning in 1967.

A second phase, the Whitehall II Study, examined the health of 10,308 civil servants aged 35 to 55, of whom two thirds were men and one third women. A long-term follow-up of study subjects from the first two phases is ongoing.

The Whitehall studies found a strong association between grade levels of civil servant employment and mortality rates from a range of causes. Men in the lowest grade (messengers, doorkeepers, etc.) had a mortality rate three times higher than that of men in the highest grade (administrators).

A striking finding from the Whitehall Studies was that the social gradient was observed for a range of different diseases: heart disease, some cancers, chronic lung disease, gastrointestinal disease, depression, suicide, sickness absence, back pain, and general feelings of ill-health.

This shows vividly the widespread impact of stress throughout our bodies. And before you ask, other factors like smoking and diet were excluded. Some have pointed to cortisol, a hormone produced by the body as a response to stress. An effect of cortisol release is a reduction in the immune system's efficacy through lymphocyte manipulation.

A study of the cortisol awakening response (the difference between cortisol levels upon awakening and thirty minutes later) further supports the significance of cortisol. Workers showed no significant difference in cortisol levels upon awakening regardless of socioeconomic position.

However, the lower employment grades showed significantly higher levels thirty minutes later, particularly if it was a workday. Researchers concluded this was due to chronic stress and its anticipation. [Kunz-Ebrect, S. R., C. Kirschbaum, M. Marmot, A. Steptoe. 2004. Differences in cortisol awakening response on work days and weekends in woman and men from the Whitehall II cohort. Psychoneuroendocrinology 29:516-528]

The Whitehall studies are far from the only research that has come to exactly the same conclusion. For example, in 2004 Schnall and Landsbergis, found that in men, there was strong, consistent evidence of an association between exposure to job strain and cardiovascular disease (CVD).

The data of the women was more sparse and less consistent. But, as for the men, most of the studies probably underestimated existing effects, researchers concluded. Other elements of causal inference, particularly biological plausibility, corroborated that job strain is a major CVD risk factor.
[2004: Belkic Karen L; Landsbergis Paul A; Schnall Peter L; Baker Dean, Is job strain a major source of cardiovascular disease risk? Scandinavian journal of work, environment & health 2004;30(2):85-128.]

My Advice
Get control over your life in any way you can, because it could prolong your life. Try to have unlimited choice, though that is not logically possible: choose where to live; when and where to take a vacation; who to go with; what hobbies you have (and, no, which television channel to watch is NOT the kind of freedom I am advocating for you). Having money to be comfortable and not work is great. Otherwise, be sure to select a job which gives you choices!

"Yes" Can Seriously Hurt You

People who are afraid of disapproval from others will say yes regardless of their true feelings, to avoid rocking the boat. The questions can range from the trivial ("Would you like a cup of coffee?") to the serious ("Can I stay at your apartment for a few weeks?").

When it comes to dealing with doctors or other caregivers, it is easy to fall into the trap of being a passive patient, afraid to say no to a suggested procedure, for instance, even though you may feel very ambivalent about it.

It's dangerous to concur sometimes! I have said elsewhere that truculent, uncooperative cancer patients (the type likely to say "Go to Hell" to their oncologist) are far more likely to survive than those that do as they are told and meekly meet their fate.

There is a big fault in reasoning here: the codependent or person who meekly acquiesces is supposing they are sparing themselves the stress of refusal. In fact, they are subjecting themselves to an even greater stress of getting something they didn't want. It's a poor trade; another example of emotional immaturity: settling for short-term comfort against ultimate long-term damage.

John W. Travis, MD, MPH, the creator of the Wellness Inventory and its parent, the Wellness Index, has this to say about the liability of meek acceptance: It's stressful. Holding in feelings of anger or frustration while smiling and saying yes causes unnecessary tension, and if you do this continually, it may erupt in physical symptoms or emotional confusion and instability.

It's confusing. Other people will read the true message in your body language, tone of voice, or energy level. They will be unsure of what you are really saying and will question your trustworthiness.

It undermines you. You erode your own self-esteem when you deny that you have insight, opinions, intuitions, and value judgments. By saying yes when you mean no, you give up your vote over what goes on in your own life. The more you deny yourself, the more you may feed feelings of low self-worth and set in motion the cycle of dishonesty/guilt/self-hatred/depression.

It disempowers others. When you assume that other people will be upset or fall apart because you say no, you are assuming they do not have the strength to hold on to their own convictions. Genuine friendship or colleagueship cannot grow from such a weak foundation. Loneliness is often the result.

The Power Of NO

Saying no can be difficult for some. John Travis suggests you work out a script for yourself, ahead of time that you can use when needed.

For example: "I know that you need help on this project, and it was great to work on it with you last year, but I have other priorities at this time that require my attention, so I will be unable to assist you. Good luck in getting the volunteers you need, and please call me again for next year." Avoid

Dr. Keith special insights

This choice thing is bigger than you can guess: In 1976, Drs. Ellen Langer and Judith Rodin studied the effects of allowing personal decision-making among nursing home residents.

They selected two floors of a nursing home. One group was told the staff was there to help them; they were not permitted to make many choices for themselves. Despite the care, 71% got worse in only 3 weeks. On the other floor where they were encouraged to make decisions for themselves, such as how to arrange furniture in their room, the residents actually improved. They were more active and happier. They were more mentally alert and more active in activities.

It was at the 18-month mark when it became really startling. Before this study, the overall death rate in that particular care facility was 25%. But in the 18 months after the experiment, the death rate among those given perceived freedom and choices dropped to only 15%, leaving the control group floor (with few perceived choices) to rise to 30% mortality.

That means being given freedom to make even simple choices, such as what TV channels to watch, whether or not, to have and care for plants, effectively halved the death rate. No medical drug can come even close to this performance in the issue of longevity. Suffocating control is quite deadly.

"The ability to sustain a sense of personal control in old age may be greatly influenced by societal factors, and this in turn may affect one's physical well being" "more successful aging -- occurs when a individual feels a sense of usefulness and purpose".

A feeling of helplessness may contribute to psychological withdrawal, disease, and death. [Langer, E., & Rodin, J., The effects of choice and enhanced personal responsibility for the aged: A field experiment in an institutional setting. JPSP, 1976, 191-198.]

Learn to Say "No"

It is little secret that stress is probably the number one killer, when viewed in the fullest sense of that phrase. Stress underlies almost every disease process in our bodies.

Take cancer survival as an example. One fascinating study I came across investigated the power of saying "No". The theory is that most cancer victims are negative about themselves and have a poor self-image; they allow themselves to be exploited; they put the needs of others before their own wants and desires. Whether consciously or not, such patients were subjecting themselves to a great deal of stress, even if it was hidden.

So the doctor who conducted this test counseled each patient to learn to say "No" to things they didn't like and didn't want to do. Start standing up for themselves emotionally. The results were remarkable. Many years later when followed up the majority of those who had learned to say "No" were still alive; those who could not stand up for themselves were dead.

According to Virginia Satir, the inventor of family therapy, one of her primary tasks was to help her clients learn to say yes when they meant yes, and no when they meant no.

It comes down to honesty. When you say YES but you mean NO, you are being dishonest with yourself and others. So it's a double whammy: the stress of not getting what you wanted plus the self-shame of enfeeblement leading to falsehood.

The emerged "vice" of co-dependence is centered around the fact that certain people will enable abusers and addicts, by agreeing with them and their behaviors, when in fact it is quite unacceptable to do so. Satir estimated that codependence afflicts over 90% of the U.S. population.

Charles Whitfield, MD, calls codependency "The disease of lost selfhood" and he considers it the root of all addictive behavior. It results from focusing too much on what is outside of yourself and thereby depending on others to define what you think, how you feel, and what you do.

apologizing. Practice your script until it sounds natural to you. The more often you speak in ways that are genuinely congruent with your own thoughts and feelings, the easier it will become.

You also need to inventory your life and look for the missed NOs! Figure out where you should have used NO, instead of a YES.

In fact, it can be good to do yourself a list and post it in view. Adapt your script, as required, for each of these areas of your life.

The thing is, although you find no unpleasant at first, it doesn't need to be a blood bath. Never apologize; it takes the position that you are wrong to refuse. Just say it politely and with good intention; assume the other person will respond in kindness. They usually do.

If he or she is very needy, you may get a negative kickback. Try to reduce contact with people like that or eliminate them altogether from your life.

The basis of joy in life is interaction and exchange, not taking instead of giving. Support only those people who support you, reciprocally. [SOURCE: Simply Well by John W. Travis, MD, & Regina Sara Ryan. Copyright 2001. Celestial Arts, Berkeley, CA.]

Faith and Meaning

Although a relatively new area of health research, studies have shown that people who are able to find meaning, or even recognize benefits, after severe adversity have better psychological adjustment, fewer recurring heart attacks, and lower mortality than those who are not.

Religion also seems to be a useful stress-coping device. Among religious people, those who report a great reliance on their faith to cope with difficult times seem to have an emotional, and potentially physical, health advantage over those who do not. For example, research has discovered that the use of religious coping is not only associated with longer life but also with lower levels of depression, lower blood pressure, and better adjustment following transplant surgery.

It's logical that a belief in some architecture behind the universe should help us cope with adversity. Those most likely to survive long years in concentration camps were the ones with faith to see them through.

It is not empowering to see the Universe as just a cold, chemical accident. Some scientists like to pretend that's the message from physics. Actually, it's the opposite. Whatever question you ask about life, if you start to investigate WHY the answer comes out as it is, and then why that? And why that? Back and back, eventually come across something akin to what Greek philosopher Aristotle called the "Prime Mover Unmoved" or Prime Cause.

It's inevitable that you will sooner or later come to something that is unanswerable, amazing, mystical and greater than we can put into words. I don't think it matters what you call it but I do think it matters that you feel its holy presence and cultivate a sense of reverence for it.

Dr. Keith special insights

Cell Phone Danger
A lot is written about the dangers of cell phones, meaning the radiation threat.

There's another danger I perceive from cell phones. They get inside your head and cause stress. Phones can mess you up. Cell phones are with you all the time and don't let up in their relentless presence.

Cell phones are a constant YES!
Living in the USA, I wonder why it is that some people feel absolutely compelled to answer the phone when it rings. It obtrudes into your time and thoughts; it will kill relaxation time; cell phones create an urgency, so that just about anything you do is speeded up, quicker than before and (mostly) quite unnecessary.

You know the old joke: most uses for a cell phone are things like "Remember to drop by the store and get an extra bottle of milk". That never used to happen. If you forgot, you forgot. Now somebody can ring you up and hassle you; or even call you a dope for forgetting.

We used to have plenty of moments of down time. Now most people think they are not alive and breathing, unless they are talking to somebody. It always idle, worthless, chatter. But people do it anyway.

Who Needs All That Stuff?
I like Jon Gordon on this, from his book "Energy Addict: 101 Physical, Mental And Spiritual Ways To Energize Your Life":

There is nothing in the user's manual to say that your phone or pager must stay on 24/7. If you don't want to be bothered during a movie, dinner, at home, or during a conversation, just shut the phone off and let your voicemail accept the call.

When you are ready to talk, simply turn your phone on, check your messages, and call people back in your time instead of theirs. You'll be amazed at how simply shutting off your phone at certain times will help you focus and increase energy.

Let's look at one important study on the benefits of belief, published in 2000 (Health Psychology). Dr Michael McCullough and his team carried out a meta analysis of studies investigating the link between faith and longevity. What they found was that people with beliefs and part of a faith group were much less likely to die in a given time frame.

Their analysis collectively involved more than 125,000 participants, over 29 studies. The length of studies included varied from a few months to two decades. To assess religious participation, subjects were asked about frequency of attendance at church or religious participation in other formats, such as praying alone or watching religious worship programs on television.

Those who were actively involved in religious and spiritual life were 30% more likely to survive. This held true, even after correcting for other factors, such as physical and mental health status, gender, race, health, behavior, and social support. [McCullough, M. E., Hoyt, W. T., Larson, D. B., Koenig, H. G., & Thoresen, C. E. (2000). Religious involvement and mortality: A meta-analytic review. Health Psychology, 19, 211-222.]

One of the studies McCulloch included in the meta analysis was carried out in California, by a Dr William Strawbridge and colleagues. Strawbridge was Adjunct Professor with the Institute for Health & Aging at the University of California, San Francisco. They followed 5200 residents of Alameda County over a period of 29 years and analyzed the relationship between frequent church attendance and death. "Frequent" attendance was defined as attending a church service at least once a week.

The risk of dying over nearly three decades was 36% lower in frequent church-goers than in those who attended infrequently. The significant difference remained, even after correcting for age, health status, social connections, and health habits. [Strawbridge WJ, Cohen RD, Shema SJ, Kaplan GA. Frequent attendance at religious services and mortality: A 28-year follow-up. Am J Public Health 1997;87:957-961].

The usual criticism of these kinds of studies (faith and health) is that the results are skewed because sick people, because of their infirmity, are less likely (less able) to attend church. But in fact both McCullough and Strawbridge went to lengths to exclude this variable factor. Strawbridge actually found that the church-going population were sicker, on the whole, than their infrequent church-going counterparts!

The conclusion of these many studies is clear: having faith and feeling close to God or some equivalent was more than just comforting; it gave meaning to life and strength to fight health issues, resulting in a longer life overall. What's more they showed it was "dose related" (like medication)! The more faith you had, the longer you tended to live.

3 | Quench Inflammation

In one word, I can tell you the number one killer disease process is - **inflammation**.

From time immemorial, medical students have been told the main characteristics of inflammation in Latin: calor, rubor, tumor, dolor. That translates to heat, redness, swelling, and pain. We are all familiar with this phenomenon; think, for example, of when you last had an infected finger from a cut.

Galen, the famous Roman doctor, was smart enough to add a fifth marker: *functio laesa*, which means loss of function. When tissues and organs are inflamed, they don't work properly. Bummer.

But what's really going on here? The answer is that inflammation is an immune response. Inflammation is what Mother Nature wants to happen: inflammation is a primary defense mechanism.

When the body is attacked by pathogens, the tissues respond with increased blood flow (hence the redness and heat); an outpouring of lymph fluid (hence the swelling); this brings white blood cells to the site and they fight with the pathogens (hence the pain). The battle royal going on in our body is what actually causes the pain.

There is a complex cascade of signaling chemicals, called inflammatory cytokines. More details on that shortly. These signaling are to mobilize defenses locally, at the site of the problem, and also throughout the body. As a result of the signaling process responding cells know where to go and what to do.

It's complex and wonderful and saves our lives every single day. We need the inflammatory process. If it failed, we would die within hours or days, as people do when their immune cells fail.

Inappropriate Inflammation

There is a problem, which is that inflammation is quite a damaging process and causes havoc in our tissues. It releases large amounts of free radicals, destruction of normal tissue, deposits of scar tissue and so-forth, though a considerable amount of repair and recovery takes place, once the invader is controlled.

If infection remains, inflammation may become chronic and linger for weeks or even years. Sometimes, chronic inflammation may persist even without significant infection - either because the inflammation response has become too sensitive or because the immune system begins to perceive some of the body's own tissues as foreign. This leads to the so-called "auto-immune diseases."

These are very damaging.

The majority of older people have some degree of low-grade inflammation and/or mild autoimmune disorders (and some have moderate or severe forms, of course). It is no wonder that chronic inflammation contributes to the aging process because it floods tissues with free radicals and promotes the destruction of normal cells.

Like most mechanisms of aging, chronic inflammation creates a vicious cycle. The aging process tends to increase the level of chronic inflammation and that, in turn, accelerates aging.

While chronic inflammation contributes to the aging of many tissues, it is particularly prominent in the aging of the cardiovascular and nervous system - the two systems most vital to our survival. Inflammation recognized as one of the key risk factors for heart disease and stroke, an even bigger risk factor than high cholesterol or homocysteine, according to some estimates. Inflammation is also viewed as a contributor to common age-related neurodegenerative diseases, such as Alzheimer's and Parkinson's.

But there are many other disease processes that have a strong inflammatory basis, including diabetes and arthritis.

How Do You Rate?

While keeping inflammation under control should be a part of anyone's comprehensive anti-aging strategy, some people are more prone to chronic inflammation than others. Hence, your first step should probably be to estimate how much inflammation you may have in your system.

Arrange to have several widely available tests: ESR, fibrinogen, and C-reactive protein (CRP). ESR (erythrocyte sedimentation rate) is a general, albeit relatively insensitive, inflammation indicator.

Fibrinogen is a part of the blood-clotting cascade: its level reflects your blood clotting capacity. Excessive clotting is an indicator of inflammation and a cardiovascular risk factor of its own.

CRP is a general inflammation indicator, but is far more sensitive than ESR. It is the primary marker for evaluating inflammation-related cardiovascular risk.

CRP levels correlate with cardiovascular risk as follows:

- Less than 1 mg/L (low risk)
- 1-3 mg/L (medium risk)
- Greater than 3 mg/L (high risk)

Additional inflammation markers known to correlate with cardiovascular risk include neopterin, matrix metalloproteinase-9 (MMP-9) and soluble intercellular adhesion molecules (sICAM).

Inflammatory Markers

Mainstream medicine has begun to recognize the importance of testing for the products of inflammation. Several articles in the prestigious *New England Journal of Medicine* have reported that these are strong predictive indicators of who will suffer a heart attack. Killer arteriosclerosis (**page 133**) remember is one of the major inflammatory diseases facing Western populations.

One of the simplest tests for hidden inflammation that should show up stealth pathogens on board, is **C-reactive protein (CRP)** or better still high-sensitivity CRP (hs-CRP). Your doctor will know this test as a cardiac profile test and you can discuss it with him or her for use as an aging marker. It is a relatively inexpensive investigation.

Levels of plasma **fibrinogen** will also tell your doctor whether you are at risk of fatal inflammatory blood clotting, due to arterial plaque rupture (**page 140**).

We also look for substances called inflammatory cytokines, which cause extensive tissue damage. Four tests that are now clinically proven to be of value as markers of inflammation are:

- Tumor necrosis factor-alpha (TNF-alpha)
- Interleukin-6
- Interleukin-1 beta
- Leukotriene B(4)

These sound a bit scary and technical but you only have to write them down and ask for them. The actual values will vary from the laboratory results and you will need someone knowledgeable to compare your results to the reference values.

As the time of this writing, at least one anti-aging laboratory is offering these tests as standard. We include them here as part of the firm belief that they should be more widely available. At present, they are outrageously expensive but supply and demand could soon see prices begin to fall.

Testing markers of inflammation in the nervous system are not as well developed but oftentimes people who have low-grade cardiovascular inflammation would have some low-grade inflammation in the nervous system and vice versa.

There are also many highly specialized tests for specific immune mediators whose levels correlate with various forms of inflammation. For example, inflammation associated with obesity often causes increased levels of the immune mediators IL-6, IL-8, and TNF-a.

If your inflammation markers are elevated, taking steps to bring them down is usually a good idea for both health and longevity. If your markers are normal but you are over forty, some basic anti-inflammatory steps may be worthwhile anyway.

The basic steps to reduce inflammation in the body include:

- **Better dental hygiene** - Low-grade gum infections are extremely common and have a major negative impact on heart disease and possibly other conditions.
- **Exercise** - Evidence indicates that regular exercise improves low-grade chronic inflammation. (It may worsen acute or active chronic inflammation, so be careful.)
- **Weight loss** - Obesity appears to increase the overall level of inflammation in the body, while bringing your weight back to the optimum (BMI 20-25) does the opposite.
- **No smoking** - Smoking floods your systems with free radicals and irritants, promoting inflammation and other forms of damage.
- **Anti-inflammatory diet** - Diet has an impact on the overall level of inflammation in your body. A number of dietary adjustments can help minimize inflammation, including the following: reducing or eliminating saturated and trans fat; increasing the intake of omega-3 fat (fish, fish oil, flaxseed oil); increasing consumption of varied multicolored fresh fruits and vegetables.

You can learn more about identifying and eliminating your own inflammatory foods in **Chapter 4** (now you understand how important it is to do this).

David Perlmutter MD, a doctor I admire greatly, has taken to using Pioglitazone ("Pio") to quell inflammation of the nervous tissue in his patients (see below).

Which of these agents, if any, are appropriate for general human anti-aging and life extension remains to be researched.

However, I have for you here some key strategies against inflammation that have proven their worth time and time again.

1. Eliminating Obesity
2. Diet Against Inflammatory Foods
3. Ozone Against Stealth Pathogens
4. General Plant Nutraceuticals With A Good Track Record.

I'll deal with each in turn.

The Missing Link Between Belly Fat and Heart Disease

OK, inflammation quickly kills you. Arteriosclerosis (or atherosclerosis), arthritis, Alzheimer's, diabetes, and even cancer are all inflammatory diseases.

Arteriosclerosis, the cause of most heart attacks and strokes, is the formal name for the process by which blood vessels become stiff, narrowed, and lined with plaque formations that forewarn of the development of blood clots. Scientists and clinicians have known for many years that it is based on inflammation.

But also, growing fat shortens your life, as everyone has been telling you! Overweight people have a higher risk of heart attacks, strokes and other problems. And people who carry their extra weight around their waist -- giving them a "beer belly" or an "apple" shape -- have the highest risk of all.

Is there anything that links these two processes together? You bet!

The dangerous fat in our bodies is belly fat, more correctly called visceral fat (Latin; viscera = guts). A team of University of Michigan Cardiovascular Center scientists have reported direct evidence of a link between inflammation around the cells of visceral fat deposits, and the artery-hardening process of atherosclerosis.

> **Overweight people have a higher risk of heart attacks, strokes and other problems.**

Belly fat harbors inflammatory chemicals (pollutants) and that's a problem. Most pesticides and synthetic chemicals are organic in nature and most dissolve in fat tissues.

You need to reduce weight to live longer. It's not the fat itself; it's what the fat does to you that kills.

The researchers also showed that a medication often given to people with diabetes can be used to calm that inflammation, and protect against further artery damage. Well, the whole of the medical "industry" only thinks in terms of drugs and making profits from disease, not actual cures.

But this one might just have a place. It's called Petoxifylline (PTX).

Drugs for Inflammation?

You will not often find me suggesting a possible drug treatment. If you do everything I say, you may never need to take drugs again! But a substance called pentoxyfillic acid (or oxypentafillic acid) has pronounced anti-inflammatory properties and could be useful to some readers.

The drug is marketed under several brand named, such as Trental, and is used to improve blood circulation and reduce clotting. Elderly patients faced with cardiopulmonary bypass surgery are far less likely to suffer the severe inflammatory after effects, if prepared with pentoxyfilline.

It also helps prevent to reactive fibrosis after radiotherapy to tumors and has been shown to prevent mitochondrial damage. It reduces inflammation and could provide useful additional therapy in any of the chronic aging diseases described above.

DOSE: the standard dose is 400 mgms three times daily (1200 mgms total). I suggest that 400 or 800 mgms, depending on body size, is fine for anti-aging anti-inflammatory properties.

WARNING: pentoxyfilline is not an anti-coagulant but *will slow blood clotting*. All to the good if you are a heart attack risk - but if you are currently taking anticoagulants, such as Coumadin, your clotting rate will have to be monitored carefully. Stroke patients require particular care, since one of the mechanisms of stroke is uncontrolled bleeding into the brain, rather than clotting. If you also supplement omega-3s, you may need to further reduce your dose of pentoxyfilline.

Talk it over with your doctor. This drug is not available over the counter.

Pioglitazone

There is lots of science coming out how "pio" benefits the widespread inflammatory processes of aging.

A range of studies have shown that it improves insulin sensitivity (biggie for anti-aging) and protects the kidney from damage due to inflammation (see item 9 in the "Speed Bumps" section on page 17). Pio markedly reduced urinary albumin, a sign of kidney damage, and reduced MCP-1 excretion (MCP-1 stands for Monocyte chemoattractant protein-1, a signaling substance that sets up inflammation by attracting certain white cells). Pio also ameliorated glomerulosclerosis and DNA microarray analysis using renal cortical tissues, several inflammatory and profibrotic genes were significantly down regulated.

Talk to your doctor about either of these drugs. It's one route to go, maybe temporarily, if your inflammatory markers are bad.

My Own Contributions

Don't forget that **ANY** food can produce inflammation in ANY person, if they are sensitized to it (food allergy, food intolerance and genetic food incompatibility). I told the whole story in the book *Diet Wise* and built a lasting international reputation on just this one phenomenon. The results I saw changing to a hypoallergenic, fresh-food, rotation diet (similar to the caveman's or Stone Age diet) was nothing short of sensational.

Miracles were an everyday occurrence (except that a miracle is when you don't know why it happened).

I cannot emphasize enough the importance of working out your own personal low-impact diet. It will keep you well for life and you'll live way longer than average. I also demonstrated on literally 10,000s of patients that even low-level residues of chemical pollutants in the body are highly inflammatory.

A recently published study showed a strong correlation between the presence of persistent pesticides in the body and the development of insulin resistance (and therefore, by inference, diabetes).

Of course, the association doesn't prove cause and effect. Let's get really scientific. There may not be cause and effect at all, or if there is, it could work the other way around. For instance, what if wheat and other grains are pesticide-ridden? If you eat lots of grains, you'll get diabetes AND pesticides in your body?

Or maybe the fact that people who have insulin resistance are already unhealthy and overloaded and therefore can do little to expel toxins (my choice)?

The researchers behind the new study, from Kyungpook National University and the University of Minnesota, felt that the action of pesticides could be contributive during the early stages of diabetes development. The study focused on the risk of pollutants from oily fish, such as methyl mercury, dioxins, and polychlorinated biphenyls (PCBs). The crucial evidence was that mere obesity did not have such a high risk factor for diabetes as obesity coupled with pesticide burden.

Now that's telling us something – but what?

What is for certain - we are all battling personal pollution on a scale unimaginable a quarter of a century ago. I first wrote about the warning signs in the early 80s and I spread the term "human canaries" in my 1986 book "Allergies: What Everyone Should Know" (actually the term was coined by my friend Ted Hamlyn).

There is no longer a secret: clean water and clean food are virtually unobtainable. Even so-called organic food is increasingly suspect, since the air and rain on which crops depend are so polluted. Most of the US's current atmospheric particulate and gas pollutants are blown in from industrial China. This is an irony to say the least, since U.S. businesses are falling over themselves to export dollars and make China a rich and dangerous enemy.

I recommend you consider an oral detoxification program. I use Garry Gordon's "Beyond Chelation" with added powdered EDTA. Plenty of Vitamin C. You can get urine test sticks, to make sure you are not scorbutic, from www.brightspot.org. Test yourself and make sure your urine checks out as bright yellow on the scale. That means you have enough C.

Dr Garry Gordon suggest a nightly oral chelation his own DMSA formula, called Heavy Detox. He also claims your skin gets rid of more mercury than fecal or urine losses and you can increase the efficiency of skin excretion by bathing with Beyond Clean (1 heaping scoop in your bathwater). Also, use EDTA soap (Beyond Soap). Add occasional Epsom Salts and/or Baking Soda to your skin rejuvenation program! see: http://www.longevityplus.com

If fish sources scare you, take capsules. Most commercial extracted fish oils are molecularly distilled and steam deodorized to remove contaminants.

Stealth Pathogens

Another major source of inflammation we call "stealth pathogens". These are microbes that hide in our bodies, invisible to the immune system, and set up chronic inflammation. In my 1980s books I referred to "smouldering viruses", though today it's clear that viruses, such as Coxsackie, Epstein-Barr, Herpes and CMV are not the only culprits. Many bacteria are guilty too—and certain parasites. But the "smouldering" part was a good choice of words, indicating these things are inflammatory and burn up the tissues.

Stealth pathogens have been discovered in urine, blood, throat swabs, brain biopsies, cerebrospinal fluid, urine, and breast milk. They are also found in patients' tumor samples with a variety of neoplastic disease, allergic disease, autoimmune disease, and neurological illnesses such as ADD, autism, depression, multiple sclerosis, schizophrenia, fibromyalgia, and chronic fatigue to name just a few.

Stealth pathogens are able to infect many different organs. The worst places to have this effect are in the brain and in the walls of our arteries. The latter sets up intractable thickening of the arteries we call atherosclerosis or, more simply, thickening of the arteries (section 10). This in turn leads to widespread body damage, due to compromised blood supply.

Stealth infections are responsible for triggering long-term inflammatory responses that many researchers believe to be responsible for Alzheimer, Atherosclerosis, Multiple Sclerosis, Rheumatoid Arthritis, and many other serious ailments.

How Do We Get Rid Of Stealth Pathogens?

Good question. They can be beaten but the answer is a comprehensive tissue clean up, not just a "remedy".

We need to tackle what's called "terrain", that is the land in which these crippling organisms set up home. If it's friendly to them, we stay sick; if we make it hostile for them, they move on!

So we want to remove all factors that favor foreign organisms living inside our bodies. That means getting rid of foods that oppress your immune systems (allergy and toxic foods, Chapter 4); getting rid of heavy metal toxins (page 192); avoiding all synthetic chemicals—not just pesticides and pollutants but all those chemicals present in manufactured foods too; and cleansing what is called the "matrix".

The Matrix In Health And Disease

Whereas so much molecular medicine is aimed at the cell, as if it were the sole seat of disease, Dr. Alfred Pischinger, then Professor of Histology and Embryology in Vienna, saw with great insight that the extracellular fluids were the key to health.

These fluids, which Pischinger called the "matrix", or ground regulation system, because it supports everything else, brings nutrition, oxygen, hormone messengers and other vital substances to the tissues and removes excretion products, toxins and the residue of old diseases.

Cells may be important but not a separate entity, because they cannot exist without being nurtured in this matrix. Reckeweg pursued Pischinger's matrix model and devized ways to use natural substances to support, clean and revitalize the extracellular matrix.

Most of the classic homeopathic remedies are still there, though used slightly differently.

Deep Tissue Cleansing

You can learn more about the important role of the matrix in health in my paradigm-busting book "Virtual Medicine": http://www.alternative-doctor.com/virtual_medicine.html

Despite a clumsy name, homotoxicology is a wonderful natural healing science. Based on homeopathy, but not quite the same thing, homotoxicology is the brain child of German doctor Hans-Heinrich Reckeweg (1905-1985). Knowing homeopathy and drawing on a vast knowledge of herbal lore and medicines, he compounded a store of remedies which trod a line between folk medicine and basic plant pharmacology.

In the course of time it has proved itself so well that tens of thousands of German doctors use it in daily practice, although it is less well known in the rest of the world. It has also been also called the German system of homeopathy, though this is slightly comical, since the original system of homeopathy was also invented by a German, Samuel Hahnemann.

Remedy Mixtures

The key variation is the use of mixtures, which classic homeopaths frown upon. But Reckeweg ignored the dogma and carried out decades of practical research, demonstrating conclusively that the formulations worked and worked well. He made compounds which would support the liver and kidneys, which would work for 'flu, diabetes, women's problems, stimulate metabolism, tone up the immune system, retard tumors, repair inflammation, act as pain-killers and so on. In other words these are function-based medicines.

The mixtures give rise to yet another name you may encounter "complex homeopathy". Not all remedies are mixtures of substances however; some are single remedies in a mixtures of several potencies (called a "chord", after the musical term for several notes sounding at once).

There are key advantages to using potency chords:

1. Deeper action
2. Fewer initial aggravations than classical dosing
3. Doses can be repeated
4. Broader spectrum of effect
5. No problems selecting the appropriate potency
6. No problems in assessing the duration or spectrum of action
7. Mixing high and low potencies produces an effect that lies somewhere in between: rapid onset (low potency) and long-lasting action (high potency). Faster action
8. Potency stages retain their own effects

Unfortunately, I cannot explain a whole science here or even suggest likely remedies. But for anti-aging, I know two which are just wonderful: *coenzyme compositum*, from HEEL and *ubichinon compositum*. Each of these mixtures is amazingly restorative.

Also in my clinic in the UK (London, Harley St), I used to give IVs with a potentized mix of all the enzymes in the Kreb's cycle. This had a great effect.

There are a number of other compounds from HEEL which will support organs and keep them vibrant and efficient until late in life. Thus there is *Hepar compositum*, to help the liver and *Solidago compositum* or *Populus compositum*, to stimulate kidney drainage. *Cerebrum comp.* is great for the aging brain and *Ovarium comp.* and *Testis comp.* may help in maintaining the vitality of sex hormones until much later in life. *Aesculus* (horse chestnut) and *Cretaegus* (hawthorn) have been known since times immemorial as cures for arterial and heart problems; now we have *Aesculus comp.* and *Cretaegus-heel*.

Triatomic Oxygen

There's one amazingly good strategy that you won't find many doctors recommending. It's ozone. I called it tri-atomic oxygen because that's its chemical formula (O_3).

Here in the US ozone is viewed as a deadly poison. The FDA frowns on it. Doctors who use it are considered quacks and criminals.

But it's widely used elsewhere in the world, by doctors in good standing, who know what they are doing. A colleague of mine, Dr. Velio Bocci, professor at Siena University (Italy) is the recognized world authority on the medical uses of ozone.

Bocci is no lightweight: He is the author of about 410 publications and monographs, mostly published in international, peer-reviewed journals including a book on Interferons (1993) and three books on oxygen-ozone therapy (2000, 2002, 2005).

In 1995, Bocci was awarded the Hans Wolff prize for innovative researches in the field of ozonetherapy. He was awarded the "Stramezzi" prize for his books on ozonetherapy by the Academy of History of Medical Art in Rome (October 2003). The Ministry of Education has nominated (May 2003) him Emeritus Professor at the Department of Physiology, University of Siena.

Basically, I go with Bocci's vast academic knowledge and ignore the idiots at the FDA.

Our interest here is summed up in a few words: **blood ozonation is a powerful and scientifically proven way to kill over 90% of stealth pathogens.**

Technique

The most effective approach is to take out some of the patient's own blood, treat it with high doses of ozone (outside the body) and then return it to the body. This is called the autohaemotherapy (or autosanguis in Germany).

A study I found from the Institute of Obstetrics & Gynaecology, Baku, Azerbaijan was very enlightening.

They were investigating infertility but tracking the effects of ozone therapy on a number of stealth pathogens, including bacteria, Chlamydia, mycoplasma, ureaplasma, toxoplasma, herpes simplex and cytomegalovirus. The organisms were successfully eliminated, up to 100% effectively.

Ozone appears to have multiple mechanisms of action.

It is widely known that ozone therapy stimulates production of immunoglobulins in the blood (IgG, IgA, IgM). But it also increases resistance of the macroorganism to microbes, improves the rheological properties (flow, viscosity and plasticity) of the tissues, stimulates the oxygen transportation mechanism of the blood and also destroys viruses with the cells.

These properties of ozone are similar to those of antibiotics, but in contrast to the latter, ozone does not have any adverse effects at therapeutic doses and microbes do not develop resistance to ozone.

In this study 56 patients displayed a range of resistant pathogens, namely:

- Chlamydiosis
- Ureaplasmosis
- Mycoplasmosis
- Gardnerellesis
- Herpes simplex
- Cytomegaloviral infection
- Toxoplasmosis
- Candida albicans
- Trichomonas

Many of these were polyinfections (more than one at once).

The patients were treated with various combinations of autohaemotherapy, rectal and vaginal insufflations, irrigation with ozonized distilled water and take-home prescriptions of ozonised distilled water by mouth.

The happy result was that 100% chlamydiosis infection was eliminated; 100% mycoplasmosis infection was eliminated; 90.9 % ureaplasmosis cured; 90.00% gardnerellesis were cured; 23% of herpes completely cured and in just over 50% the levels were reduced by half; 83.33% of cytomegaloviral infection there was complete cure; 17.65% of toxoplasmosis was cured and in 35% of cases the level was reduced by half.

That's pretty impressive and shows how effective ozone is against notorious stealth pathogens.

Insufflation

If you don't have access to IV ozone because of local regulations, you can get great benefit from rectal (or vaginal) insufflations of ozone (gas passed into the rectum, where it is readily and painlessly absorbed).

The most common infectious agents reduced or eliminated by rectal ozone are Entamoeba histolytica, Giardia lamblia, Campylobacter jejuni, Clostridium difficile, Shigella spp., Neisseria gonorrhoeae, Chlamydia trachomatis, Treponema pallidum, HSV, Mycoplasma hominis, Ureaplasma urealyticum, group B streptococci, HAV, HBV, etc., and in patients with clinical AIDS also CMV, Cryptosporidium spp, Isospora spp, Mycobacterium avium-intracellular (MAI), HIV, etc.

Rectal ozone is effective for the treatment of sexually acquired proctitis most commonly from N. gonorrhoea, HSV, and C. trachomatis, less commonly U. urealyticum, C. albicans, T vaginalis, T pallidum, H. ducreyi, Calymmatobacterium (formerly Donovania) granulomatis, HBV, HIV, CMV, EBV, and human papillomavirus; as well as sexually acquired proctocolitis, enterocolitis, and enteritis due to Campylobacter spp, Shigella spp, E. histolytica, G. lamblia, and others.

Prostaglandins

A Swedish doctor, Ulf von Euler, first discovered this important group of inflammatory body substances in the early 1930s. He discovered semen caused experimental smooth muscle samples to contract. It was thought the active ingredient, obviously an irritant, originated from the prostate gland, thus the term prostaglandin was coined.

In the 1940s, another Swedish doctor, Sune Bergstrom, took the research further and discovered prostaglandins were derived from fatty acids, identifying two types, which he called PGE1 and PGE2. He also learned prostaglandins were found in many tissues, not just semen.

In 1971, a UK research student, Jim Willis, showed that the way aspirin and other non-steroidal anti-inflammatory drugs (NSAIDs) worked was by blocking the synthesis of prostaglandins.

Then in 1973 Dr. David Horrobin injected himself with prolactin developing premenstrual type symptoms: bloating, irritability and depression. He later showed that prostaglandin E1 (PGE1) opposed this unpleasant effect. Basically, E1 is the "good guy" (soothing) and E2 is the "baddy", causing irritation and hence inflammation.

Since then, we have learned that prostaglandins are hormone-like substances playing a role in many body functions, some of which appear to cause inflammation, blood clotting and other tissue damage, while others appear to be beneficial. It's likely the two types interact, keeping each other in check and providing the balance needed for perfect health.

PGE1 is an extremely active substance with a whole range of properties, including inhibiting inflammation, preventing platelets from sticking together, vasodilatation, inhibiting cholesterol production, and stimulating underactive brown adipose tissue (the kind that burns off excess fat).

On the other hand, the 2-series prostaglandins (derived from arachidonic acid, an omega-6) produce a reddening of the skin and tissue swelling.

There are several other players in this game: leukotrienes and thromboxanes. The latter name should tell you that these inflammatory substances increase the risk of blood clotting and hence the threat of heart disease.

Both PGE1 and PGE2 are vital to optimum health – an imbalance appears to have adverse effects on the skin, cardio-vascular, reproductive and immune systems. The last is of special importance to allergies.

Omega-3 essential fatty acids, DHA and EPA, lead to increased production of "good" prostaglandin E1, which counters the bad inflammatory prostaglandin E2. For more than two decades, we have known the important role of prostaglandin imbalance in promoting tissue damage. Fish oils and flax seed (linseed) oil are your sources of omega-3s.

DHEA and antioxidants such as vitamin E, carnitine (acetyl-N-carnitine) and n-acetyl-cysteine (NAC) also lower pro-inflammatory cytokines.

If your cytokines or CRP is raised, you need to avoid foods, which contain pro-inflammatory ingredients. Arachidonic acid is an omega-6 fatty acid and leads to prostaglandin E2. You need to eat less red meat, especially organ meats. You also need to cut out foods with a high glycemic index: breads, cakes, pastries, sweets, fruit juice, etc. and since sugar is pro-inflammatory, it should be eliminated or at least significantly reduced.

Instead these foods will reduce your inflammatory cytokines: our old friends oily fish, fresh fruit, vegetables, salads, nuts and oatmeal.

4 | Your Personal Survival Diet

How To Live 100 Years

Those of you who have read my book Diet Wise will be familiar with this historic tale, from Renaissance Italy…

The central character was a Venetian nobleman called Luigi Cornaro. He was born in 1467, which makes him a contemporary of Michelangelo Buonarotti and Leonardo da Vinci, who were busy with numerous others, creating world-shaking art in Florence.

A typical nobleman of the day, Cornaro squandered his considerable fortune on high living, especially food and drink. Unfortunately, his constitution was rather weak and he was racked with symptoms, including indigestion and gout, attended by an almost continuous fever and thirst. He was getting steadily worse.

Cornaro would probably have died by the age of forty, as most people did in those days, but he was lucky. One of his physicians told him, in no uncertain terms, that he had better sober up his lifestyle – or call the undertakers.

Shocked by the possibility of imminent death, Cornaro decided the smart thing to do was to listen to the doctor's advice (which for once was sound and holistic). He began to experiment and found that he felt better if he ate less and avoided certain foods that seemed to upset his constitution.

In fact, Cornaro was the first person on record to work out his own **Custom Fit Diet**. He was pretty smart and realized that the foods he liked or craved were not necessarily the best for him. More on that in Chapter 4.

Cornaro found that he did not tolerate fish, pork, melons and other fruits, salad (though he doesn't say what ingredients), rough wines and pastry. Surprisingly, the foods he could tolerate included meats and certain choice wines. He liked an egg, bread and soup.

Eat less and eat right was his basic formula. In his case, he was able to tolerate twelve ounces of food daily and fourteen ounces of decent wine. Within a year he was fully healed, zestful and enjoying life. The years rolled by, fifty, sixty, seventy, eighty! Apart from a couple of episodes, he remained well. One setback was a serious coach accident at the age of seventy, which almost cost him his life.

Cornaro was dragged from the wreck with many bruises, a dislocated arm and a broken leg. The doctors wanted to bleed him (as if he wasn't shocked enough). Cornaro wisely refused and relied on his own diet management formula to restore his damaged limbs.

It worked

The second near fatality occurred when he broke his diet, at the insistence of concerned relatives. They believed he should fatten himself up, to maintain his strength. As a result of continued nagging, he decided to up his rations to fourteen ounces of food a day and sixteen ounces of wine. Within a week he was peevish and quarreling with all comers.

By the tenth day he was seized with a violent pain in his side, which lasted over twenty two hours, before being succeeded by a serious fever, which lasted for thirty-five days. Cornaro abandoned the changes and soon recovered.

In fact, he went on to live an exceptionally long and healthy life. At the amazing age of eighty-three he published his first treatise, entitled: *The Sure and Certain Method of Attaining a Long and Healthful Life*. The English translation went through numerous editions. He wrote three more pamphlets on the same subject, composed at the ages of eighty-six, ninety-one and ninety-five respectively. Luigi Cornaro finally died, serene and dignified, at the age of ninety-eight.

What was remarkable about Cornaro's achievement was the age in which he lived. The average life expectancy of the time was under forty years. To live beyond three score years and ten was almost unheard of, never mind reaching two years short of one hundred. Cornaro had clearly made a major discovery in the field of disease and health; you would think the medicos of the day would be won over and want to pass on the good news, but they ignored Cornaro's remarkable diet experiments.

I resurrected it for you in Diet Wise and the book explains in splendid detail how to carry out the same dietetic experiments Cornaro did. He had never heard of inflammatory foods or personal nutrigenomics (see later in this section) but he sure proved it worked to human benefit.

Get a copy of the book "Diet Wise" here:

http://www.dietwisebook.com

Inflammatory Foods

Not many people understand just how stressful foods can be. Because we think of foods as nourishing—something our bodies need—the fact that many foods are toxic and damaging gets overlooked. Yet "toxic food syndrome" is real and is here.

I'm not talking about poisonous foods we all avoid; I'm talking about everyday foods we all eat at some time or another. The shocking truth is that many foods are not well tolerated. But because it's a personal or idiosyncratic thing, doctors are not paying enough attention.

This is where I first entered the anti-aging arena, over three decades ago. I was putting people on allergy exclusion diets, avoiding the common stressor foods, and I found something remarkable: almost every single patient who went on my "Stone Age Diet" (Man's natural diet) felt and looked 10 – 15 years younger!

There were a lot of delighted faces around my office! Family and friends were being electrified and asking "You look terrific; what are you taking?" The irony was that it was not something added but something taken away that produced the rush of vitality and brain clarity.

I learned in a very vivid way that foods can be profoundly negative effects; even supposedly healthy whole foods, like whole grain wheat, milk and eggs. Not everyone is affected by the same foods and so we used to call it food allergy. It wasn't classic allergy but very much the same outcome: avoid the allergen and feel good!

The term food "intolerance" was introduced, to try to get round the problem that true immune mechanisms were often hard or impossible to demonstrate in most cases. Nowadays, we know that most of this food intolerance phenomenon comes from minor variations in genes that we call SNIPs (see page 61). The important point is that badly tolerated foods, let's call them stress foods (or toxic foods!) can be highly inflammatory.

If the idea of food being biologically stressful seems strange to you, consider the last time you over-indulged at the table to the point of wishing you hadn't: did you feel ill, bloated, sweating, maybe abdominal pain, pounding pulse, drained of energy, slumped in a chair hardly able to move? If that isn't stress caused by food, what is?

> **Knowing and avoiding inflammatory foods will lead you to devise your very own Personal Survival Diet.**

But the inflammatory food phenomenon I'm going to teach you about is much more subtle than this. They disguise themselves almost completely from view, like terrorist sleepers. In fact, the chances are high that you are eating one or more stress substances *every day,* without realizing it.

You are going to need my book Diet Wise, which will tell you what to do about this phenomenon. Get yourself a copy and work through it conscientiously and I promise you it will make you look and feel years younger. I knew then and I know now that aging can be reversed, not merely halted.

We are talking now about your number one ticket to a long and healthy life.

http://www.dietwisebook.com

Knowing and avoiding inflammatory foods will lead you to devise your very own Personal Survival Diet. Because of the variable tolerance of foods, no "one-size-fits-all" diet can possibly work for everyone. Forget the Atkins Plan, the South Beach Diet, the Blood Group Diet, the X-diet, the Y-diet, the Z-diet.

They may be best-sellers but what you never hear is that every fashionable diet actually makes some people ill. The authors never tell you that; it would hurt their sales.

Even vegetarianism is toxic for many. The number one offending food that people do not tolerate is wheat (actually, the whole botanical family of grains or cereals). Number two is dairy produce (milk, cheese, cream, yoghourt, ice cream etc). These are the two foods that vegetarians rely on heavily as dietary staples and may explain why so many vegetarians *look* rather pasty and unhealthy, no matter how they describe themselves. Far more people react to wheat and/or milk than meats and so would not suit being vegetarian.

My stand is a contentious one: any diet that works well for an individual does so because they have inadvertently avoided stress foods. For instance, if milk is one of your toxic foods, a low-fat diet will effectively eliminate dairy products from your diet and you would feel great. Any improvement, such as weight loss and disappearance of migraine or arthritis, would be attributable to milk avoidance, not low fat at all.

Similarly, many people are said to be sensitive to gluten but are not: they improve because of wheat intolerance; they can eat other gluten foods with no ill effect (rye, barley, oats).

Personalized Nutrigenomics

Things have progressed rapidly since my pioneer days; we now have a whole new understanding of how this toxic food phenomenon comes about. Some of it is true allergy; some of it biochemical or pharmaceutical intolerances such as with a caffeine "allergy"; some of it is enzyme deficiency and so on.

But it really all boils down to one thing, your genetic makeup. Nutrigenomics is a term we apply to the study of how genetic variations affect our metabolism and the way we use and process nutrients, including vitamins and minerals.

There is one important principle to grasp, which good alternative doctors have always known but conventional medics refuse to even consider - *we are all different*.

Orthodox medicine is based on the concept of averages, even though not one single person alive today is "average." There are too many variables for this to hypothesis to work. It is wrong to ignore these numerous differences and just pretend we are all the same. It hurts patients and invalidates therapies. Drugs become dangerous for some people, when they cannot detoxify it to something safer, like everyone else. Daily doses accumulate, until fatal levels are reached in the blood. That's the story of Vioxx and numerous other disasters.

The thing is, while it's true we all share a lot of DNA, nobody is the same as anyone else. You remember all the fuss when the genome project was announced? It was going to solve everything. We'd learn at last the true nature of diseases.

Then it emerged that humans have only around 20,000 genes: about the same as an earthworm and less than some plants! Although they haven't admitted it yet, this throws the whole DNA hypothesis on its head. Add to that the discovery that RNA, the supposed subservient "messenger" molecule, can switch genes on and off and the whole landscape has got busted!

What has emerged is a whole new fascinating science!

SNPs (pronounced "snips")

This term stands for single nucleotide polymorphisms. A fiery sounding name! But it just means slightly altered slices of code in a gene. There are 4 amino bases stuck to the sugar chains in DNA, let's call them ACTG. So a little run could go: TTCTGAAC. But some human beings, maybe even just one person, could have: TGCTGAAC. Not quite the same.

The difference is probably not enough to kill the person but it might mean they cannot manufacture as much of a certain enzyme as the rest of the population. Let's say it's the enzyme to break down toxic levels of compound "X". That means this individual will be extremely intolerant of compound "X". It makes them very sick, while everybody else can cope with it.

Example: Let's Look at Codeine

The liver converts codeine into morphine using the enzyme CYP2D6, a process that causes pain relief in most people. However, genetic differences in some people cause either too much or too little of the enzyme to be produced. Too little will render codeine ineffective; too much will create unpleasant reactions, such as excessive sedation, respiratory depression, severe constipation and other side effects attributable to excess morphine.

Over-production only occurs in about 4% of Caucasian North Americans, prevalence is much higher in people from Greece and Portugal (10%), Saudi Arabia (20%) and Ethiopia (30%), while under-production happens in about 6 – 10% of Caucasians, 3 – 6% of Mexican-Americans, 2 – 5% of African-Americans and about 1% of Asians.

These racial differences should alert you right away to the fact these differences stem from minor genetic variants, which is exactly what I have been saying. But it isn't quite that simple. Certain medications can also affect one's CYP2D6 activity. The enzyme's production is inhibited, for example, by diphenhydramine (Banadryl) and quinidine (Duraquin, Quinaglute, Dura-tabs or Quinidex).

So someone who produces too little CYP2D6 and is slow to eliminate quinidine might find no benefit at all from codeine, if they concurrently take Duraquin! There again we are showing just how individual each of us is.

I hope this excursion in molecular biology and genetics enables you to understand how complex it can be and how very important it is for efficacy of medication and safety to work within these principles. Ignoring these individual differences renders conventional medicine toxic and dangerous.

That's why over 100,000 people a year die of correctly prescribed medicines in the US alone.

If you or a loved one chooses to take prescription meds, take half the dose first time, to see how you tolerate it (unless it's an emergency). NEVER take more than the dose suggested, unless you are sure you can tolerate it.

Vitamins Alter Gene Expression

In 2008 a milestone paper from Berkeley University was published, showing just how vital proper nutrients are, including much-maligned vitamins and minerals [Published online before print June 3, 2008, doi: 10.1073/pnas.0802813105 PNAS June 10, 2008 vol. 105 no. 23 8055-8060]

As Nicholas Marini, the lead author of the Berkeley paper said: physicians will often prescribe drugs to "cure" many rare and potentially fatal metabolic defects caused by mutations in critical enzymes. But those affected by these metabolic diseases are people with two bad copies of an essential enzyme. Many others may be walking around with only one bad gene, or two copies of slightly defective genes, throwing their enzyme levels off slightly and causing subtle effects that also could be eliminated with vitamin supplements.

"Our studies have convinced us that there is a lot of variation in the population in these enzymes, and a lot of it affects function, and a lot of it is responsive to vitamins," Marini said. "I wouldn't be surprised if everybody is going to require a different optimal dose of vitamins based on their genetic makeup, based upon the kind of variance they are harboring in vitamin-dependent enzymes."

Food Pharmaceuticals

Now add to what you have just learned the complex pharmacology of foods and you will see the dangers right away. Foods contain many complex chemicals and if these cannot be properly metabolized, then the individual is at risk when eating those foods.

Doctors will never discover the real problem, because they are not looking for it. Instead, the patient will be classed as a faker or psychiatric case; because they keep claiming that certain foods or places make them feel sick. "Unscientific nonsense", says the doctor.

Patient stays sick, or maybe mysteriously dies (remember Heath Ledger?).

What's wrong with the "bad gene" theory?

Let me counter the "bad" gene hypothesis. This is something orthodox medicine considers to be an absolute and permanent affliction. People who recover from such diseases are simply not acknowledged; they cannot have recovered, therefore they didn't, is a sort of blind credo that doctors stumble along with, ignoring facts that are plain to all the world who sees with an unbiased eye.

The best reaction such an event might get is "spontaneous remission". There are no "spontaneous" recoveries. **They all have a reason and a valid scientific explanation.** It's just that sometimes we don't know what the underlying science is.

> **You can turn off all your bad genes if you go about this the right way.**

The fact that such recoveries sometimes they lie outside conventional science, means that orthodox doctors will say "There is no explanation". I would say differently.

The trouble with the "bad gene" story is that it assumes we are helpless. Already that is yesterday's science. In recent years it has emerged more and more strongly that it's possible to manipulate genetic disorders very favorably. This can be done in the same generation, the same individual, that the genetic effect manifests.

This alone is startling and makes nonsense of Darwinian evolution as taking place by mere chance, as the "natural selection" theory requires.

I'm not espousing intelligent design here but thinking more of Lamarckian evolution. Jean-Baptiste Lamarck (Jean-Baptiste Pierre Antoine de Monet, Chevalier de Lamarck, if you like fancy names!) was a French scientist, adopted by the Soviet Union for doctrinaire reasons and ignored in the West for equally doctrinaire reasons. He argued that developed traits which benefitted the organism could be passed onto the offspring (Darwinian evolution says that can't happen; the unsuitable offspring, without the beneficial trait, die out is how it works).

Most scientists still think that harmful mutations are disfavored by evolution but logically that can only apply to mutations that affect reproductive fitness. Mutations that affect our health in later years are not efficiently removed by evolution and may remain in our genome forever.

Now we know that genes, although "fixed" structurally, are very plastic when it comes to manifesting or what we call "expressing" their traits.

The whole movement of environmental allergies and chemical sensitivity of which I was among the founders in the 70s and 80s was really based on the precept that the environment was the real cause, not the person's genetic makeup.

Geneticists began to talk of partial or incomplete expression of traits, caused by environmental factors. So, as I said in my 1986 book, what does it matter? It all comes down to environmental factors: that's where we should look! What turns genes on and off?

Those factors are the REAL cause of diseases.

Foods do it with remarkable ease. You need to get your own diet perfected and stick to it. You can turn off all your bad genes if you go about this the right way. That's how to live longer, despite what you were born with in your make up.

5 | Carbohydrate Control

Are You Serious About Staying Out Of A Nursing Home For Your Last 20 Years On Earth?
I hope so.

A July 2007 study once again pointed to the importance of carbohydrate metabolism and the way in which persistently raised insulin levels trigger degenerative diseases, notably diabetes. In fact, you will find me saying often in my writing that diabetes is a kind of mirror for the aging process. If you are unlucky enough to contract diabetes, the whole aging cycle moves very much quicker with you than for a normal person.

You do NOT want raised insulin levels, at any cost.

We already know from laboratory studies that keeping insulin unnaturally low extends the lifespan of a nematode worm called *Caenorhabditis elegans* and fruit flies quite significantly. Both creatures are used to study aging mechanisms. The big question remains: does this apply to mammals?

This interesting trial centers on mice bred to have low insulin signaling in their brains; they simply did not secrete the hormone, even in the presence of raised blood glucose. In fact even when put on a high glycemic index diet (rich in carbs), they still did not secrete much insulin. This is very different from the normal response, which is that insulin levels go up when blood glucose levels go up.

Eventually, on a chronic high refined sugary carb diet, the body tires of the whole process, and more and more insulin pours into the blood, but the cells no longer listen and blood glucose levels are not brought down.

We call this state **insulin resistance**! The next stage is diabetes, a result of control mechanisms that are dysfunctional. You die young. The interesting thing is that once diabetes is established, even while keeping blood glucose levels low by means of drugs or insulin injections, that the massive degenerative process takes place anyway.

It's bad news all the way.

You have probably already learned that keeping insulin levels down is one way to live longer. Now genetically-engineered mice that have a lowered insulin response have a 17% longer lifespan, despite being push-fed on carbs. That just rams it home yet again. In human terms, avoiding carbohydrates and managing your insulin levels within safe limits would mean, according to this trial, an extra 12.75 years. That's more than a whole decade of bonus living!

These results, the investigators write, "point to the brain as the site where reduced insulin-like signaling can have a consistent effect to extend mammalian lifespan."

They also concluded that the findings support the idea that the reduction of circulating insulin through moderate daily exercise, calorie restriction, and weight loss may also increase lifespan by keeping insulin signaling in the brain low.

"This study provides a new explanation of why it's good to exercise and not eat too much," lead investigator Morris White, PhD, a Howard Hughes Medical Institute investigator in Children's Division of Endocrinology at Children's Hospital, said in a news release. "It has less to do with how we look, and more to do with a healthy brain, especially in old age."

Interestingly, human centenarians display increased peripheral insulin sensitivity and reduced circulating insulin concentrations. That's probably not because they lived to 100 but why they lived that long.

[1Science. 2007;317:369–372.]

Low Carbs Help Weight Control

There are other good reasons to keep your carbohydrate intake within bounds. Another bang up-to-date study (July 24, 2007) compared the health benefits of high and low glycemic diets in respect of weight loss and blood lipid profiles. This was what is called a Cochrane database survey, meaning a re-working of a number of studies already filed in the Cochrane database.

Same story. Avoiding carbs (low glycemic index foods) was more beneficial in terms of overall weight loss and improving total cholesterol and those tricky low density lipoproteins. Not surprisingly, the effect was more pronounced for obese subjects.

It's just as Buddha Atkins pronounced! Just please remember Robert Atkins was actually very late in the sequence. Low carb diets have been going around since the 19th century. The first was William Banting; in fact Banting became a verb and society debutantes and flappers in the 1920s used to say "No cake for me, I'm Banting!" In the 1940s we had the Air Force Diet.

Then in the 1970s my great mentor Richard Mackarness brought out a book called *"Eat Fat and Grow Slim"*. I don't think it sold terrifically well, because the title seems to be too unbelievable. But if he'd called it the "Dr Atkins Diet Revolution", I expect he would have made many millions of dollars!

[Cochrane Database Syst Rev. Published online July 18, 2007]

What should you do?
- Eat no refined carbohydrates.

- Eat whole complex carbohydrates sparingly. There is PLENTY of sugar and carbohydrates in foods like peas, beans, carrots and root vegetables. Use mashed butternut squash instead of potato and mashed cauliflower instead of rice for a curry dish.

- Eat frequent small meals, rather than single heavy meals. Nibble something every 90 minutes or so: just nuts, an apple or even cheese, whatever. We call this grazing (like a cow) and it's far healthier.

- Exercise some. It's hard to set standards but the minimum, if you are serious about staying out of a nursing home for your last 20 years on Earth, is 30- 40 minutes of vigorous walking 3 times a week. It will do nothing for your weight or body mass index but it WILL make you more insulin sensitive and help lower blood glucose.

Remember Nature (God) designed us as hunter-gatherers. Make as if you are walking along in the forest and eating food as you go. Keep moving! Keep nibbling! That just about sums it up. No heavy meals followed by slobbing out on the sofa.

Are You At Risk?
Do this today…

I want you to take a tape measure and measure your waist. Don't cheat or breathe in! Let it hang out. Then measure the largest circumference of your hips and note down the two figures. Your waist should be LESS than your hips. Preferably a couple of inches less.

The reason is that yet another study has suggested that waist-to-hip ratio is much more sensitive than body mass index (BMI) at predicting risk of subsequent coronary disease.

Writing in an early online edition of Circulation, Dr Dexter Canoy (University of Cambridge, UK) and colleagues report that increased abdominal obesity — measured in terms of waist-to-hip ratio, was more "consistently and strongly" predictive of coronary heart disease (CHD) than BMI among men and women participating in the European Prospective Investigation Into Cancer and Nutrition in Norfolk (EPIC-NORFOLK) study.

"In our study, in men who were obese and had lower waist-to-hip ratios, their rates of CHD tended to be slightly lower than if they had high waist-to-hip ratios." Coney said. "But in women, at all levels of BMI, waist-to-hip ratios were strongly predictive of heart disease."

The study showed that even if we take into account habits like smoking, alcohol intake, or sedentary lifestyle, and we take into account what we already know are important predictors of CHD such as hypertension and dyslipidemia, you will still have an excess risk of a heart attack, if you have a higher than 1.0 waist-to-hip ratio.

Waist circumference alone was also a fair predictor of CHD events, but not nearly as accurate as taking the ratio of waist and hips together. Other recent studies have also shown that this is the best predictive measure we have.

A Big Bum Protects!
Basically, for every increase of roughly 6.5 cm (2.5 inches) in hip circumference for men, and for roughly 9 cm (3.5 inches) in women, risk of developing CHD was reduced by 20%.

That's not to say people should develop a big hip circumference to protect themselves from risk, but for any body size, those with bigger hips tended to be associated with lower risk.

The importance of this new direction in health is this: we know overweight and obesity is a risk factor. But, if the overweight individual has larger hips than waist, the risk is actually somewhat attenuated.

Conversely, if you are of a normal weight, or maybe only mildly overweight; you should not be smug. Formerly, doctors would pat you on the head and say "Don't worry; you're fine."

Well now we know that *if your waist-to-hip ratio is bad, you are in danger, even if your weight is a healthy average*. That's different to what you have learned over the years, I'm sure. But you need to let it sink in. I want you to live much longer than average and now I can no longer say just keep your weight in trim.

I have to say keep that waistline inside your hipline! To be very exact (if you have a calculator handy), your risk can be assessed as follows:

MEN	WOMEN
0.95 or less (low)	0.80 or less (low)
0.96- 1.0 (moderate risk)	0.81- 0.85 (moderate risk)
over 1.0 (high)	over 0.85 (high)

[Canoy D, Boekholdt SM, Wareham N, et al. Body fat distribution and risk of coronary heart disease in men and women in the European Prospective Investigation Into Cancer and Nutrition in Norfolk Cohort. A population-based prospective study. Circulation 2007; DOI: 10.1161/CIRCULATIONAHA.106.673756. Available at: http://www.circ.ahajournals.org.]

Obesity
Obesity remains close to the top of conditions that will shorten your life. Insurance actuaries are very clear on how the percentage risk of death rises with every pound overweight; they are very exact about calculating the value of human life and the likelihood of an expensive payout. Pay attention to this scientific cynicism; they can turn your chances of survival into an exact statistic!

Refined carbohydrates make you gain weight inexorably. Most people find losing weight easy when avoiding carbohydrate, without starving themselves or feeling hungry. This diet theme has been in circulation for over a century, as I said.

Atkins has been probably the most famous and successful low carbo plan of all time; the acclaim is simple – it works, despite everything the critics throw at it. Now the late Doctor Atkins has spawned a whole rash of "me too" plans, such as the South Beach Diet.

World-class health author Leslie Kenton has recently reworked the theme yet again, in a fine book called "The X Factor Diet" (Vermillion 2002) and Barry Sears "The Zone" is essentially that same life-saving information. Learn it and do it.

Low carbo eating is gentler and more successful than low calorie plans. Everything you eat has calories. Whereas there are hundreds of foods that score zero on the carbohydrate monitor and can be eaten extensively. Where I disagree with Atkins is the way he *pushed* fats. That's not necessary.

Metabolic Syndrome

Our understanding of disordered blood glucose control advanced considerably in 1988 when Dr Gerald Reaven of Stanford University published a paper describing what he called "Syndrome X". A syndrome in medicine means a group of symptoms appearing together, as a characteristic pattern, which is repeatedly encountered.

> **Most people find losing weight easy when avoiding carbohydrate, without starving themselves or feeling hungry.**

In this case, the syndrome consists of five features: obesity, insulin resistance, high blood pressure, high serum triglyceride levels (bad fat) and low HDL (good cholesterol). Dr Reaven had no idea what caused this group of symptoms to occur together, so he named it "Syndrome X".

Notice that patients with Syndrome X do not have the dangerously raised glucose levels of diabetes. However, they do have insulin resistance and higher than normal levels of circulating glucose. The high level of insulin stimulates the kidneys to re-absorb sodium, which in turn results in a tendency to hypertension. Dr Reaven believes that half of all hypertensive's have insulin resistance. No-one needs to be told of the dangers of high blood pressure.

Raised triglycerides, along with raised LDL (bad cholesterol), combined with lowered HDL are disturbing. These changes in blood fats denote a major increase in the risk of arterial degenerative disease.

Unfortunately, hyperinsulinism also reduces the level of blood enzymes which prevent or dissolve blood clots. Thus, along with the undesirable changes in blood fats comes a sinister increase in the likelihood of thrombosis, making the risk of heart attack or stroke far greater than for healthy individuals.

Nowadays syndrome "X" has a proper name; we call it the Metabolic Syndrome. You may also hear it referred to as Reaven's syndrome and CHAOS in Australia.

Many people are unaware that they have Metabolic Syndrome, even though the American Heart Association estimates that 20-25% of the adult population of the U.S. suffers from this disorder – between 58 and 73 million men and women.

Today, we have a fuller definition of Metabolic Syndrome, which is characterized by having at least three of the following symptoms:

- Insulin Resistance (when the body can't absorb blood sugar or insulin properly)
- Abdominal fat – in men this means a 40 inch waist or larger, in women 35 inches or larger
- High blood sugar levels – at least 110 milligrams per deciliter (mg/dL) after fasting
- High triglycerides – at least 150 mg/dL in the blood stream
- High LDL "bad" cholesterol
- Low HDL "good" cholesterol – less than 40 mg/dL
- Pro-thrombotic state (e.g. high fibrinogen or plasminogen activator inhibitor in the blood)
- Blood pressure of 130/85 mmHg or higher

The American Heart Association states that the "underlying causes of Metabolic Syndrome are being overweight, physical inactivity and genetic factors."

There is an increased link between Metabolic Syndrome and other diseases, such as polycystic ovarian syndrome (PCOS) in women and prostate cancer in men.

Inflammation Again

The exact mechanisms of the complex pathways of Metabolic Syndrome are not yet completely known. Most patients who suffer it are older, obese, sedentary, and have a degree of insulin resistance. Stress can also be a contributing factor (see section 1, cortisol).

There is debate regarding whether obesity or insulin resistance is the cause of the metabolic syndrome or if they are both perhaps consequences of a more far-reaching metabolic derangement. A number of markers of systemic inflammation, including C-reactive protein, are often increased, as are fibrinogen, interleukin 6 (IL-6), Tumor necrosis factor-alpha (TNFα), and others (see Chapter 4). Some have pointed to a variety of causes including increased uric acid levels caused by dietary fructose.

In my view, the inflammatory aspect of this condition is what makes it so deadly. Once again, inflammation equals early death. No debate.

Diabetes

The basic conditions enumerated by Reaven (obesity, insulin resistance, high blood pressure, high serum triglyceride levels and low HDL) can be referred to as "pre-diabetic". Sooner or later, left untreated, the condition is going to worsen and turn into full-blown diabetes.

Diabetes itself has emerged as something of an auto-immune disease (body attacking itself), with inflammation as one of its core features.

I look on diabetes as an (unwanted) overview on the process of aging. Much of the degeneration in the arteries, heart, brain, and eyes seen with diabetes is the same as that attributable to aging. But it takes place much faster in a diabetic patient. The life expectancy of an individual with diabetes is therefore considerably below average.

Here we refer to type II diabetes or "late onset" diabetes. As its name suggests, this is mainly what affects older individuals. It is a direct result of collapsed carbohydrate regulation. Whereas type I diabetes is caused by the failure of the pancreas to secrete adequate insulin, in type II there is **too much** insulin. The two conditions are fundamentally different. In the type II condition the body has become refractory to insulin, simply not responding to regulation as it should. Thus, despite high levels of insulin, glucose increases to unacceptable levels in the blood. Be sure you understand: *untreated diabetes is a fatal disease process*.

The tragedy is that successful regulation of blood insulin and glucose levels do not protect you from the degenerative damage. That's why drug control is a waste of time. You need to settle down that inflammation and for that my Diet Wise program is crucial (see **Chapter 4**).

The many complications of diabetes can be summed up as follows: arteriosclerosis (leading to increased risk of heart disease, stroke and gangrene of the lower limbs), early dementia, impotence, eye damage leading to blindness, poor kidney performance, nerve damage, resulting in numbness and paralysis of the limbs, skin sores, carbuncles, ulcers and poor wound healing.

Be aware then: you do not want to develop diabetes at any stage of life. Beware what you eat!

Laboratory Testing
In the old days the main test was tasting the urine to see if sugar is detectable: hence the term diabetes mellitus (sweet tasting)! Fortunately, things are more scientific these days! We are more interested in blood levels. These days we tend to use a measure called the hemoglobin A1c test -- also called HbA1c, or glycated hemoglobin test, or glycohemoglobin -- an important blood test used to determine how well diabetes is being controlled, because it provides an average of blood sugar levels over a six to 12 week period.

Doctors will insist on isolated blood glucose measurements, though these can be very misleading, even when fasting, and random samples are worse than useless.

More helpful is the **glucose tolerance test**. The patient fasts overnight and then, after a loading drink of 50 grams of glucose, blood samples are taken hourly. Usually this is continued for 2-3 hours but far better is to go 4 hours.

The diagnostic sign is that the glucose level goes high (over 180) and stays high or is very sluggish at returning to pre-test levels. This means the cells are not utilizing the glucose properly, either through frank lack of insulin, or due to insulin resistance.

Guidance values are as follows:

TIME	Normal test range (mg/dL)
Fasting	70- 110
30 minutes	110- 170
1 hour	120- 170
2 hours	70- 120
3 hours	70- 120

At least two of the recordings must be abnormal (high) to diagnose diabetes.

Hyperinsulinaemia is mainly diagnosed by sophisticated blood tests, showing abnormally high insulin levels without proportionately raised glucose levels. Blood insulin levels are difficult to measure and so not done routinely. The GTT is much more valuable if insulin is measured concurrent with the glucose levels.

> **Be aware: you do not want to develop diabetes at any stage of life. Beware what you eat!**

The so-called **insulin tolerance** test means giving an injection of insulin to a fasting patient (one unit per kilogram of body weight) and taking repeated blood glucose samples every three minutes for a quarter of an hour. Insulin resistance is diagnosed if the blood glucose falls by less than 50% of the fasting level in those 15 minutes. The test is not safe to perform if the fasting glucose is less than 120 mg/dL.

Hospital doctors and internists prefer to measure blood hemoglobin AIC or glycosylated hemoglobin. That tells them much more accurately what long-term changes in blood levels of glucose have been like. Normal levels range up to 7%. Above 7% is bad, above 10% very bad and above 12% is dangerous, and means very poor glucose control. Experts recommend repeating this test every 3- 6 months once diabetes has been established.

What You Can Do
By the time you have developed diabetes, you need help from a qualified and skilled doctor. But the only aim of the ordinary physician is to control the disease by keeping the blood glucose levels within normal limits.

You will be offered drugs, which increase insulin secretion (such as the sulphonyl ureas) or a different kind of drug metformin, which increases the body's sensitivity to its own insulin. This simplistic approach does not go nearly far enough for you. It is far better to tackle the causes.

You can do a great deal to avoid disordered carbohydrate metabolism, or help yourself towards a recovery, if you have understood the origins of the problem. First and most obvious is to drastically curtail the amount of carbohydrate in your diet. Avoid all sugar, flour, and "white foods". What carbs you do eat, take only as whole-grain products.

Exercise and weight control are vital at all stages of life but particularly if you are in the high risk zone (50 plus). All knowledgeable practitioners agree these two decrease insulin resistance significantly. Both also help in reducing hypertension. Do not even consider medication for blood pressure, unless all lifestyle changes fail – drugs will merely mask the problem and not eliminate the cause.

Dr Reaven restricts carbohydrate and replaces it with mono and polyunsaturated fats, such as olive oil and fish oils. These increase insulin sensitivity and help reduce triglycerides and LDL. However, some care is required, omega-3 fats (fish and flax oil) are known to potentially impair insulin levels and increase blood glucose. This adverse effect may be avoided by adding vitamin E (400 IU daily) to the regime. The omega-6 fatty acids (evening primrose oil, star flower, borage) has insulin-like properties and also increases sensitivity to insulin but without affecting bad blood fats.

Supplements

Top of the list is chromium, aka "glucose tolerance factor"! Take at least 400 mcg daily.

Next comes DHEA, which lowers insulin levels and also protects organs, particularly the kidneys, against damage due to high blood glucose levels. See pages 121-122 for advice on dosing.

Next comes magnesium. A consensus panel of doctors in the America Diabetes Association agreed that magnesium deficiency may play a role in developing insulin resistance, carbohydrate intolerance and hypertension. Pay attention: it is not often that conventional doctors recommend nutrient solutions! Take 350 mgm a day or more.

Vitamins B3, B6 and C are also vital. Deficiencies have shown up as insulin resistance. Take 100-1,000 mgm of B3, 50-100 mgm of B6 and 2 grammes of vitamin C daily, alone or as part of your health formula.

Alpha lipoic acid, a star-quality supplement steadily climbing to the top of the anti-aging league table, apart from being a powerful antioxidant has also been shown to improve insulin action. You need 200-400 mgms daily.

Fiber

Fiber has a number of beneficial effects on metabolism. One of the most important is supporting probiotic life. But almost equally important is helping to dampen down surges of blood glucose. By slowing down the absorption of carbohydrate foods, fiber is one of the main regulatory substances for insulin.

Dense carbohydrates, the complex type found in whole grains, are slow to digest and slow to absorb, so do not cause major spikes in blood levels of carbs that are so characteristic of refined and processed foods. Whole grains, if you can tolerate them, are a good food source because they boast fiber and complex carbs.

Aloe Vera

You probably know about the marvellous healing plant *Aloe vera*. It's been used in healing since 3,500 ago in Egypt. But you may not know it can help support balanced blood sugar.

A double-blind study in the journal Phytomedicine split 78 people into two groups. One group was given aloe vera daily. The other was not. After just six weeks, those taking aloe were better able to balance their normal blood sugar by 43%! [Bunyapraphatsara N., et al. "Antidiabetic activity of Aloe vera L. juice II. Clinical trial in diabetes mellitus patients in combination with glibenclamide." Phytomedicine. 1996;3,(3):245-248].

The control group that didn't take aloe had an average blood sugar increase of 2.4%.

In another study from 2006, Japanese researchers conducted a clinical trial of 70 people. They found that daily intake of aloe vera helped reduce levels of fasting blood sugar and glycated hemoglobin. Glycated hemoglobin is a measurement of how high your blood sugar has averaged over the last 90 days. [Tanaka, M, et al. "Identification of Five Phytosterols from Aloe Vera Gel as Anti-diabetic Compounds." Biological and Pharmaceutical Bulletin. July 2006;29(7):1418-22].

Products

An excellent range of products to try are the Univera products, especially Xperia, and Aloe Gold. Prime, from the same range, also has a good reputation for helping shed 10-12 lbs. painlessly, as well as providing DHEA, 7-Keto DHEA, vitamin B6, vitamin B12, alpha lipoic acid, n-acetyl cystine (NAC) and acetyl l-carnitine. I take it myself, not that I would pass as obese.

Univera have just brought out an even more sensational glucose control product, called **Level-G**. The supportive science is very impressive indeed. I just haven't had chance to get supplies and try it yet!

To learn more email for a catalogue: **admin@informed-wellness.com**

You can also try complex homeopathic formulas, especially the HEEL range referred to on page 51.

Italian suppliers of the same type of medications are Guna and US distributors Deseret Biologicals also get my vote.

Here are some useful addresses:

Guna Worldwide:
GUNA S.p.a.
Via Palmanova 71
20132 MILANO - ITALY
Phone: +0039 02-280181
http://www.guna.it

Guna USA:
GUNA Inc.
3724 Crescent Court West
Whitehall, PA 18052, USA
Phone: (484) 223-3500
www.gunainc.com

Deseret Biologicals
469 Parkland Dr Sandy, UT 84070
801-563-7448
desbio.com

6 | Detox – Stemming the chemical blizzard

OK, we've looked at diet from two different angles (inflammatory foods and carbohydrate control). Eating right is the single most important thing you can do to give yourself a happy and vibrant life, right up to your last days.

But I also teach that good food and a "balanced" diet is not enough for us to stay healthy. Maybe it was once, back in Neolithic times. Archeological evidence shows superb and healthy skeletons from our ancestors.

But today we are fighting a very toxic environment, loaded with free radicals and oxidizing agents. It is simply stupid and very UN-scientific to say that what Nature gave us is enough. It isn't; not any more. We need extra nutritional support for de-toxing; a LOT of support!

Our bodies have to de-toxify what I call a "chemical blizzard" that we are exposed to. There are literally millions of synthetic chemicals, of which around 70,000 are in constant production at any one time. Most of these are such strange combinations of atoms, not found in Nature that our bodies simply don't know how to deal with them. We lack the metabolic pathways.

Human Chemical Contamination

The medical literature confirms that many foreign and toxic chemicals are increasingly contaminating the blood of the American population. In a 2003 CDC study on 2500 volunteers (representative of the U.S. population), all of the 116 man-made pollutants being investigated were found in the blood of these volunteers. A respected news report of this study stated:

"Two independent teams of scientists report that bodily fluids carry chemical cocktails that include toxic metals, artificial hormones, and ingredients of plastics, flame retardants, pesticides, herbicides, and disinfectants."

In 2007, 'The Faroes Statement' was a landmark scientific declaration on the dangerous accumulation of many chemical toxicants within the human body. In particular, the statement addresses pollutants with significant adverse hormonal and developmental effects.

The Faroes Statement (published by world-renowned experts in immunology, biochemistry, neonatology, genetics, developmental toxicology and other scientific disciplines) included the following:

"Part of the new insight derives from numerous animal studies on fetal programming being responsible for reproductive, immunological, neuro-behavioural, cardiovascular, and endocrine dysfunctions and diseases, as well as certain cancers and obesity. These adverse effects have been linked to chemical pollutants at realistic human exposure levels similar to those occurring from environmental sources."

Certain chemicals can be detected in a person's blood, fat and other tissues, in spite of no interim contact with that particular toxic substance for many years. For example, Vietnam veterans who served in the US Army Chemical Corps (a unit that sprayed Agent Orange) are readily distinguishable from others in the population due to much higher dioxin levels in their blood, decades after the Vietnam conflict.

There are also growing concerns of the genetic damage caused by many of the pollutants with which the U.S. population is extensively contaminated. Some children now have a significantly higher risk of the development of cancer, due to DNA damage produced by pollutant chemical exposures, especially in early fetal growth before they were born.

There is now a clear link between the presence in humans of persistent organic pollutants (POPs) and the subsequent higher risk of diabetes, especially from contamination with organo-chlorine chemicals.

The Liver

Our liver is the principle detox organ that tries to keep us safe. But there is a limit to what the poor old liver can accomplish, without giving it support and assistance.

This is where nutritional supplements become important: we can't hope to match the necessary levels just by eating a healthy diet. We need to add more, a lot more, but we need to supplement intelligently.

Back in the 70s and 80s there was a fashion for mega-nutrient therapy, which meant taking lots of everything "to be sure". This was a rash strategy because then, as now, we don't know all there is to know about how vitamins and minerals interact with each other. Taking too much of one thing can be detrimental to the status of another. For example excess zinc can create a relative copper shortage.

A better idea was to try and figure it out and come up with the best combination strategies. Linus Pauling suggested the name "orthomolecular" dosing. *Ortho-* means good, straight and healthy, as in orthopaedics, good bones. Notice the correct spelling with ae, not orthopedics, which would be just straight feet (from Latin *pedis* meaning foot). Orthopaedics is not old-fashioned, it is the correct spelling, going back to its roots: ortho-, straight + the Greek *paes*, child = the practice, literally, of straightening the child.

To practice orthomolecular medicine requires a very comprehensive understanding of physiology and disease conditions. It is little understood and even less practiced. I cannot claim to exhibit it here because it's also a personal thing, different for everybody. But I can give you some good pointers that will enable you do choose sensible supplements and sensible doses.

Never mind the idiot doctors who scoff at what they call expensive urine.

Understanding Detox Pathways

This section might seem a little bit technical; it is. But as in most aspects of life, the more you understand the better choices you can make.

The way I explain it, isn't so difficult!

Basically, in dealing with foreign substances in the body, our liver and mitochondria in the cells have two principle pathways of clearing them. Detoxing isn't quite the right word, though it's passed around a lot. The correct term is *biotransformation* and is more accurate than detoxing because **biotransformation, sometimes, changes the substance into something even more toxic!**

Biotransformation takes place in two stages, Phase I and Phase II.

Phase I is simple; it is the process of adding oxygen, hydrogen or hydroxyl ions, or taking away chlorine atoms, to neutralize the toxic nature of the substance by transforming it chemically.

There is a whole family of enzymes to do this, called the cytochrome P-450 system. I wouldn't bother to try and memorize that name. But it is the subject of intense scientific study, as the ravages of our chemicalized world become more and more apparent, even to mainstream medical scientists.

> **Biotransformation, sometimes, changes the substance into something even more toxic!**

Phase I biotransformation needs certain micronutrients to make it work, notably B2, B3, B6, B12 and folate, magnesium, and iron. We call these helper substances "co-factors".

Phase 2 biotransformation is the chemical process of linking the toxin with another atom group, such as a sulfate or methyl group, to make it water-soluble. That way the chemical can be excreted by the kidneys or passed into the bowel as a constituent of bile, directly from the liver.

We call this linking process "conjugation". The most important molecule in our bodies for this purpose is glutathione. The trouble is every toxic molecule gotten rid of results in the loss of a glutathione molecule. So in battling our toxic world we need lashings of glutathione.

It doesn't work well to take it by mouth (though claims for new liposomal delivery are interesting in this regard). We need to take the precursors of glutathione: N-acetyl cysteine (NAC), cysteine, methionine and alpha lipoic acid are the best.

One of the most significant enzymes for Phase 2 is sulfite oxidase, by which the sulfur-containing molecules in drugs and foods are safely metabolized. It is also the process by which the body eliminates the sulfite food additives used to preserve many foods and drugs.

Those with a poorly functioning sulfoxidation detoxification pathway are more sensitive to sulfur-containing drugs and foods containing sulfur or sulfite additives.

This can be especially important for asthmatics, who may react to these additives with life-threatening bronchospasm. Molybdenum is essential for the function of sulfite oxidase, so make sure you take some, especially if you are sulfite sensitive. Nobody knows how much but I suggest 100 mcg.

Toxic Intermediates

That's all there is to chemical "detoxing" or biotransformation!

But it isn't quite so simple, of course. For one thing, many of the intermediate chemicals can be quite toxic in their own right, which is why the term detox isn't right. Some of these metabolites, as they are known, can cause extensive inflammatory and oxidative damage.

So we need lashings of good antioxidants to be present at all times. Lots of carotenes (orange-yellow), anthocyanicins (blue-green), vitamins C and E, selenium, copper, zinc, manganese; and liver protectors, such as coenzyme Q10, cruciferous vegetables and silymarin (milk thistle). Silymarin is many times more potent in antioxidant activity than vitamin E and vitamin C, which is why it has become a famous "liver protector".

Another problem is that, especially in the presence of nutrient deficiency or substances which slow Phase 1 (grapefruit juice, antihistamines and capsicums can all do that), the process may bottleneck. If that happens, side pathways open up and this can be very dangerous. Epoxides, for example, are unwanted Phase 1 metabolites that can cause DNA damage and lead to cancer.

That's probably the pathway which allows toxic synthetic chemicals to be carcinogenic.

Drug taking, Candida, and alcohol are some of the many substances which will overload the biotransformation pathways. Watch out for them and live the clean life as much as you can.

This bottlenecking can also be a problem if Phase 1 works fine but Phase 2 doesn't. Some people are born that way; it's a gene fault. These people are hypersensitive to chemicals, "allergic to the 21st century", because they accumulate toxins very easily and can't get rid of them.

Phase 3

A third aspect of biotransformation has been suggested. I first noticed it using complex homeopathics (homotoxicology, see **Chapter 3**) back in the 1980s. Others have reported it and now mainstream scientists are talking about it.

It's the fact that sometimes, in an overload situation; cells cannot seem to pump out toxins. They lack enough energy to pump chemicals against the gradient. It's a vicious circle because the chemical, which is reducing the cell's energy, may be the one it wants most to get rid of.

This energy-dependent efflux pump (to use its fancy name) is called the *antiporter activity* of a cell.

Two genes encoding antiporter activity have been described: the multi-drug resistance gene 1 (MDR1) and multi-drug resistance gene 2 (MDR2). The MDR1 gene product is responsible for drug resistance of many cancer cells, and is normally found in epithelial cells in the liver, kidney, pancreas, small and large intestine, brain, and testes. MDR2 activity is expressed primarily in the liver, and may play a role similar to that of intestinal MDR1 for liver detoxification enzymes.

What To Do

OK, you want to get on top of this detox (biotransformation) thing: what do you do?

Step 1 - Seek A Competent Health Specialist

First of all, you must get a work up from a competent health specialist. Detoxing (I'll stick with that term for now) can be dangerous if done carelessly. It mobilizes toxic gunk from all over your body. If you are not careful you'll end up depositing bad stuff in organs like your brain, instead of getting it out of your body altogether.

Dr. Sherry A. Rogers, M.D., in her seminal book **Detoxify or Die,** underlines the seriousness of the matter. "The protocol is to first be sure your mineral levels and detox pathways are healthy. Have your doctor write a prescription for the RBC Minerals and Heavy Metals, as well as for the Detoxification Capability Panel (MetaMetrix). There are other suitable mixes, of course. Just make sure you get the right ones.

To mobilize mercury from 'safe' storage in tissues and bring it out into the blood stream, can force it into the kidneys, brain, or other organs if your detox capability is not strong enough to complete the job and flush it out into the urine. People have died because of failure to assess detox capability before oral chelation.

If you are already ill or fighting a disease, it may not be appropriate for you to do a heavy metal detoxification. I have personally had patients come in who took ill-advised detoxes with enthusiastic but ignorant amateurs and ended up on a stretcher. Be warned!

Today I unreservedly recommend Intestinal Metal detox (IMD) from Christopher Shade. More of that in the Miscellaneous Factors, which is Chapter 14.

Step 2 - Get Rid Of Ongoing Sources
It's no good going in for any kind of detox program if you don't first get rid of the source of pollution. So, for example, you cannot detox from mercury while you still have silver amalgam fillings in your mouth.

Several oral health problems can reduce the effectiveness of a mercury detoxification program. You need to work with a good biological dentist to improve your oral health status. Phone the I.A.O.M.T. (International Academy of Oral Medicine and Toxicology) at 863-420-6373 to find an accredited dentist in your area. You will also find a database of mercury-free dentists at www.dentalwellness4u.com.

As Tom McGuire DDS says in his book *Mercury Detoxification: The Natural Way to Remove Mercury From Your Body*: "There is a direct relationship between a healthy mouth and a successful mercury detoxification program. By decreasing the effectiveness of the immune system, the above oral infections can interfere with the body's ability to remove harmful metals and other toxins.

"In addition, some of the symptoms directly related to oral disease can mimic those of chronic mercury poisoning. Thus, you could be successfully eliminating mercury and still exhibit symptoms that imitate those of chronic mercury poisoning; but are actually being caused by an oral infection or infections.

"You can be certain that unless you identify, treat, and eliminate all of these oral health issues you may not get the results from your detoxification program that you'd hoped for. This doesn't mean that you need to wait to begin your detoxification program until you have eliminated all of your oral health problems.

"On the contrary, the reverse is also true and mercury can interfere with the body's ability to deal with these oral health conditions, such as making gum disease more difficult to treat."

Don't forget, as I revealed in my own book "Virtual Medicine" dental and especially gum disease is the number one marker for who will die of cardiovascular disease. Hidden dental infections can be lethal!

Step 3 - Clean Up Your Environment
On the same elimination theme, get rid of all unnecessary chemicals in your surroundings. With very few exceptions, soaps, sun blocks, skin creams, hand lotions, deodorants, shampoos, cosmetics, perfumes, insect repellents, etc. all contains toxins.

Don't be naïve; all these schlocky substances get absorbed through your skin. Up to 90% absorbed and they can do considerable harm to your liver, kidneys and brain.

Also, be careful what you use around the house. Avoid pesticides and other garden poisons; aerosols such as air "fresheners"; solvents.

Step 4 - Improve Your Diet, Get Rid Of Toxic Foods

That's a theme I keep coming back to, over and over. But there is no way round it. Reduce your chemical load by eating organic as much as you can.

More importantly, as I have emphasized over and over, is what you get rid of, not what you eat. Avoid all manufactured foods, as a lifelong habit, and work through the Diet Wise program referred to on **page 58**.

The one thing I want you to ADD is fiber. There is no question; it helps in the binding of toxic compounds, and helps get them excreted. Most toxins are removed via the bowel. You want them to stay in the bowel and not get re-absorbed. Fiber is critical for this.

4. Drink Enough Water To Help Your Kidneys

After the liver, skin (sweat) and the kidneys are our two main detox organs. Both need water. Filtered is better than what comes in plastic bottles, loaded with BPA and phthalates.

I recommend at least an activated carbon filter. A good reverse osmosis system is better, since it takes out solids and chemicals. You can tell simply if you have enough water on board: your urine will be very pale or colorless.

> **Filtered water is better than what comes in plastic bottles, loaded with BPA and phthalates.**

Some people advise against drinking much with meals. It is said, to dilute digestive enzymes. I do not subscribe to this view, which goes against experience. The first rush of water in the stomach is quickly removed by simple absorption. The rest of the fluid stays in the bowel lumen and the final adjustments to water intake are made upon reaching the colon.

Saunas

Our skin is our largest elimination organ; in fact it's our largest organ, period. Sweat contains measurable amounts of toxins, safely removed from the tissues. Logic says sweat more!

The basic philosophy of attempting to enhance human detoxification has been used for thousands of years. Commonly known examples are Roman and Turkish baths, Scandinavian saunas, and North American native sweat lodges.

But we can get methodical about this. Some years ago a new program emerged and it is supported by doctors like, who know their holistic and overload facts; it's called "thermal chamber depuration".

What this means is low temperature saunas. A typical sauna is anywhere from 160 – 180 degrees F. That's hot enough to be dangerous and no-one should spend more than 15 minutes at a time in a hot sauna without taking a cooling plunge. But a "thermal chamber" is just a term we use for safer temperatures, around 100 – 120 degrees F. That means you can stay there longer and sweat more.

Depuration is a fancy name for washing away toxins. It's used in the shellfish trade, where clams, oysters etc are subjected to running water, to swill away toxins. It's not to describe an extraction process; just the way that the toxins will hop into the water as it goes by and be carried off (low-tech explanation).

You can add vigorous exercise to your regimen before you go into the low temperature sauna. That will increase sweating.

These days, far infrared saunas are best for this process. Typical temperatures are around 100-120 degrees F. You can stay in up to 45 minutes or even an hour, once you have become accustomed to using this type of sauna.

I would suggest you do it 30 minutes daily, as part of a serious detox regime, over the space of 2 weeks. But if you are not on an intense program, 45 minutes once or twice a week should be OK.

Remember, the more you sweat, the more pollutants come out of your skin. That's good. But do shower off afterwards, before you re-absorb them. Also, treat a sauna that's used often as a potentially polluted zone.

7 | Nutritional Supplements Against Aging

My Top 12 *Non-Hormonal* Anti-Aging Supplements

Remember, all good health measures are anti-aging! Sugar is particularly deadly for brain function and contributes to beta amyloid deposits. Ronald Reagan's notorious sweet tooth may have led to his Alzheimer's. Also bad are excess alcohol, tobacco, saturated fats, and stress. Take exercise regularly. The following supplements can be considered for a scientifically based anti-aging regime, without resorting to hormones.

Anti-aging in this sense means looking after yourself, staying alert mentally and full of vitality. It doesn't necessarily mean living longer.

1. L-Carnosine

Although carnosine has been known for about a century, its anti-aging properties have only been extensively studied during the past few years. It may turn out to be the greatest anti-ager of all. High concentrations of carnosine are present in long-lived cells such as in nerve tissues. The concentration of carnosine in muscles correlates with maximum lifespan, a fact that makes it a promising biomarker of aging. Unlike most antioxidants, which work by prevention, carnosine protects AFTER free radicals have been released. One of the cardinal anti-aging affects in the body is glycosylation, which leads to decay of protein function. Carnosine blocks this process. It also blocks amyloid production, the substance found in the brains of Alzheimer's patients. Other properties emerging are its apparent anti-cancer effects, toxic metal binder, and immune booster.

DOSE: 500 mgms. daily. Best with vitamin E, 200-400 IU daily.

2. Trimethyl Glycine (TMG)

TMG protects the youthful methylation process in our metabolism. Published research shows that methylation/TMG can lower dangerous plasma homocysteine levels, thus reducing the risk of heart disease and stroke. It helps the integrity of nerve fibers and so may improve Alzheimer's and Parkinson's disease. It protects against liver damage from alcohol and other dangers. Finally, it protects DNA and so may slow cell aging.

DOSE: 500 -2,000 mgms. daily. It works better with co-factors B6, B12 and folic acid.

3. Gingko Biloba

Extract of the tree Gingko Biloba has been used by the Chinese for 2800 years. It is now well recognized as an important brain food and anti-oxidant and improves mental function in people of all ages. It quenches free radicals and improves neurotransmission, thus protecting circulation and enhancing memory. Even the Orthodox Journal of the American Medical Association reported it to be well tolerated and effective. It protects against Parkinsonism, Alzheimer's and other dementias.

DOSE: 50-100 mgms active ingredient. Look for products with less than 2 ppm of the toxic gingkolic acid (European limits set at 5 ppm maximum).

4. S-ADENOSYL METHIONINE (SAMe, pronounced Sammy)

A derivative of important methionine, SAMe is widely distributed in the tissues of young healthy adults. But with aging and sickness, it is depleted, leading to further deterioration. SAMe is needed for the body to metabolize efficiently, for neuronal regeneration and the synthesis of energy through ATP, the basic energy molecule. It may help prevent or reverse liver damage (alcohol, viruses and chemical pollution). It can help with ME and other fatigue states.

SAMe may be the safest, fastest acting anti-depressant available and is widely prescribed in Europe for that purpose. Additionally, with betaine, it works as a scientifically-proven liver protective.

DOSE: 200-800 mgms daily. Best taken on an empty stomach, with water.

5. N-Acetyl-Cysteine (NAC)

L-cysteine is an important sulphur-containing amino acid. Others, taurine and methionine protect and nourish the liver. The form N-acetyl-cysteine is more readily absorbed and is a powerful antioxidant and anti-viral. This could be important when we recognize more and more the damaging effects of "stealth viruses". It also helps boost glutathione levels, which is one of the most important brain detox substances of all.

DOSE: 500-1000 mgms daily. Note: Take plenty of extra vitamin C at the same time, to prevent it being oxidized and rapidly destroyed in the body (3 times as much vitamin C as N-acetyl-cysteine is recommended).

6. Phosphatidyl Choline (And Phosphatidylserine)

No point in living to a great age if your brain doesn't travel along with you. Phosphatidyl choline, from lecithin, is an important protector for phospho-lipid cell membranes in the brain. These are the ones most easily damaged by free radicals.

We get it in our diet, in vegetables (especially cauliflower and lettuce), whole grains, liver, and soy. It also comes in lecithin (containing 10-20% phosphatidyl choline) in grains, legumes, meat, and egg yolks. But, we need more, to be on the safe side.

Most of these remarks apply also to phosphatidylserine, a phosopho-lipid. It is found in fish, green leafy vegetables, soybeans, and rice. Over 3,000 published research papers and more than 60 clinical trials have established that phosphatidylserine can rejuvenate your brain cell membranes and cognitive function.

Both these compounds are valuable to memory and mood, mental clarity, concentration, alertness and focus. Got to keep those grey cells going!

DOSE: 500 mgms daily of phosphatidyl choline/100 mgms daily phosphatidylserine.

7. Coenzyme-Q-10
This vitamin-like substance (also known as ubiquinone) was discovered in 1957. Since then a deluge of scientific papers have attested to its ability to strengthen the immune system, lower blood pressure, prevent heart attacks, counter obesity and slow aging. Studies in mice show it increases their life span by 25%. CoQ10 is found in all cells, where it is responsible for the manufacture of ATP, the basic energy molecule. It is now being said that if CoQ10 levels drop by 25%, cancer is probable.

On a personal note, when I took co-Q-10 and selenium simultaneously, my hair started to grow back - dark hairs!

DOSE: 100-200 mgms daily. It is plentiful in heart, meat, kidney and eggs, and to a lesser extent soybean, wheat, alfalfa, and rice bran.

8. Boron
The pivotal role of boron in bone metabolism has made it clear that it is protective against osteoporosis and therefore vital to a long and happy life, especially for women. More women die from complications of a fracture of the femur in the USA than of breast cancer. Researches also concluded that countries with lower boron levels in the soil had much more arthritis. It works best in conjunction with magnesium and other co-factors.

DOSE: 3 mgms daily, coupled with 300-400 mgms of magnesium.

9. Alpha-Lipoic Acid
The subject of intensive current research, this may be the most important antioxidant of all in protecting the brain and neurological tissues from damage. Alpha-lipoic acid has the unique ability to pass into the brain, where it helps regeneration of other antioxidants, such as vitamin C and E and glutathione. It is also a good chelator and may protect against Alzheimer's by removing toxic metals, which generate damaging free radicals. It is both fat and water soluble, which means it is easily absorbed from the gut.

DOSE: 60-80 mgms.

10. Vitamin E
Now I need to bring your attention to a report published in the Journal of the American Medical Association (Jan 23rd 2008). It says (yet again) that vitamin E is good for you. It stops aging decline.

This time an unequivocal 60% greater odds of physical decline in people with the lowest blood levels of vitamin E, compared to people with the highest levels of vitamin E.

The study in question randomly selected almost 700 adults over age 65 from an ongoing longitudinal study in Tuscany, Italy. Blood tests were reviewed to ascertain vitamin levels and it also reviewed data from physical function exams completed at the start of the study and at the three-year follow-up.

After adjusting the data to account for other factors that could contribute to physical decline, such as smoking or a lack of physical activity, the researchers found two factors were significantly associated with a greater chance of experiencing physical decline -- age and low levels of vitamin E.

Low levels of B vitamins, vitamin D and iron didn't increase the odds of physical decline, apparently.

It has always been known that vitamin E could help prevent serious illness, such as heart disease or Alzheimer's. However, a recent scandal of junk science tried to discredit this and other antioxidant vitamins and it was suddenly announced that taking these vitamins can damage your health! The media rode the story like they were dancing on the grave of natural and complementary medicine.

Well, here's the real truth. You won't hear this on CNN, of course.

The RDA for vitamin E is absurdly low and has a great deal to do with the current atrocious state of US health. At 30 IU (about 20 mgs), the "recommendation" will kill you. You need 200-400 IUs. I see no point in taking more. It's allopathic think to suppose that if some is good, more is better.

Don't forget you must take the mixed form. The "normal" vitamin E (alpha-tocopherol) alone is not protective and probably unhealthy. You need gamma-tocopherol too.

11. Vitamin D

Talk about a back runner coming to the fore and winning the race! Since the rickets problem was "solved", nobody has paid too much attention to vitamin D. Doctors think it helps calcium for bones and that's the end of it.

Not a bit! Vitamin D is one of the most powerful of all vitamins with a variety of effects that prevent the decay process of aging.

We now know that vitamin D can reduce or prevent heart disease, several cancers, cardiovascular disease, autoimmune disorders, psoriasis, diabetes, psychosis, and respiratory infections including colds and flu.

Researchers proved that people with the highest levels of vitamin D had a 43 percent lower rate of heart disease. If that's not enough, another study in the American Journal of Clinical Nutrition found that vitamin D can decrease your risk of cancer by up to 77%.

Two other recent meta-analyses (in which data from multiple studies is combined) conducted by the Moores Cancer Center at the University of California at San Diego and colleagues suggested that raising blood levels of vitamin D could prevent one-half of the cases of breast cancer and two-thirds of the cases of colorectal cancer in the U.S.

If a drug could do that, doctors would somersault with delight to have it at their disposal.

The sad truth is doctors continue to turn to statin drugs when treating their patients. I would never trust my life to satins and the fake science their surrounds their marketing.

For one thing, statins dangerously depress levels of coeznymeQ10. That alone is likely to put you in your grave years early. Remember statins "science" is about whether they prevent strokes or heart attack. No discussion ever of whether they kill you in other ways!

Moreover, statins come with side effects that can be dangerous in their own right. Some of the most common side effects are muscle aches, fatigue, joint pain, and impotence. Fatigue can be so bad that you can't exercise. And, if you do exercise, you gain weight and go into the decay cycle.

But what's worse, you can also develop a condition called rhabdomyolysis. This is when your muscle cells begin to break down. You become sore and weak. But you may have other symptoms, like nausea or an abnormal heart rate. It can develop into kidney failure and early death.

Avoid statins (and doctor) if you want to live a long and healthy life.

What Dose?
I recommend you aim for a minimum of 2,000 I.U. of vitamin D3 per day (must be D3, to impact your immune system). If your level tests low, take 4,000-5,000 I.U. a day from a variety of sources. There is no worry of toxicity at this level.

You can get enough vitamin D from sunlight but this is unreliable, unless you live half-naked in the tropics! Factors that decrease the body's ability to make vitamin D include dark skin, heredity, obesity and certain medications, including some anti-seizure drugs and, of course, sunblocks.

We can get vitamin D through foods such as fortified milk and cereals as well as eggs, salmon, tuna and mackerel, but the amounts are not nearly sufficient to lift blood concentrations to optimal levels.

12. Essential Fatty Acids
Almost the same status as vitamins, essential fatty acids are vital for tiptop body and mind function. So-called omega 3s and omega 6s have different effects. You need both. Plant sources, such as borage and evening primrose, provide omega-6s and fish oils provide omega-3s. Studies show that eating plenty of fish reduces inflammatory chemicals and leads to better health and more mental clarity, with less chance of Alzheimer's. Didn't your mother tell you eating fish is good for the brain?

DOSE: 500-2,000 mgms. Food sources - fish, starflower, borage, evening primrose and flax seeds.

How Good Are Omega-3s?
Very good. They protect your arteries and brain.

But here's surprise news. They also protect very significantly against cancer and that's one of the "speed bumps" we seriously have to avoid, in order to ensure a long and happy life.

Fish Oil And Cancer Amazing Study

Swedish scientists recently published an important paper on the positive impact of omega-3 fatty acids, found mainly in fish oil, on a certain type of childhood cancer called neuroblastoma (Gleissman 2010). These Karolinska Institute scientists had previously shown that DHA (the most unsaturated form of fatty acid in fish oil) could cause apoptosis (i.e., programmed cell death) in cancer cells.

They have now extended their work to experimental animals, showing that fish oil supplementation caused either stabilization or actual regression of tumors in these animals. They state, DHA "is a promising new agent for cancer treatment and prevention of minimal residual disease" (ibid). I will show their conclusions have relevance to a broader range of adult cancers.

The paper encompasses two parts: one on treatment, the other on prevention. In the prevention half, they gave DHA as a food supplement to rats before the animals were implanted with human neuroblastoma cells. (Because they lack a thymus, the rats in question are unable to reject tissue from a foreign species.)

In the treatment half of the study, athymic rats that already had established neuroblastomas were force fed DHA daily and their tumor growth and DHA levels were then monitored. The authors concluded "untreated control animals developed progressive disease, whereas treatment with DHA resulted in stable disease or partial response." The response depending on the dose of DHA.

But DHA also considerably slowed the development of the tumors. There appears to be a very special relationship between DHA and nerve tissue. For instance, a deficiency of DHA will lead to delayed neural development. In this case the tumors were "profoundly deficient in DHA," whereas the level of the competing omega-6 fatty acid arachidonic acid (AA) is increased.

This suggested to the authors that "an imbalance between omega-3 and omega-6 fatty acids may serve as an adaptation mechanism in nervous system tumors." Logically, then, one might expect the addition of DHA to slow or even stop the growth of the tumors.

Anything that helps treat or prevent cancer, one of the biggest speed bumps on the way to successful aging, is great news for us. That's why omega-3s are one of my star "down and dirty dozen".

Eating more fatty fish seems, even more than ever, a prudent thing to do. Children, too, should be encouraged to increase their DHA intake through fatty fish consumption. However, with the Gulf of Mexico oil spill, finding good sources of non-contaminated fish is likely to become even more difficult than it already has been. High quality supplements of DHA and EPA may therefore be the best solution for most readers. For vegetarians, getting sufficient amounts of DHA and EPA can be a challenge. The best sources are walnuts, flaxseeds and flaxseed oil, olive oil, canola (rapeseed) oil, and avocado. DHA supplements derived from microalgae, not fish, are also readily available.

Now here's another surprise…

Iodine, The Orphan Nutrient

At all times iodine is critical for life, yet it is often forgotten. I consider it a powerful anti-ager. Iodine is essential for sound function of the thyroid gland, which in turn regulates our metabolism and energy. You do not want to be deficient in iodine.

The trouble is, it's one of the most widespread nutritional deficiencies in the world. According to WHO, in 2007, nearly 2 billion individuals had insufficient iodine intake, a third being of school age. ... Thus iodine deficiency, as the single greatest preventable cause of mental retardation, is an important public-health problem. [The Lancet (12 July 2008). "Iodine deficiency—way to go yet"/The Lancet 372 (9633): 88.]

To make matters worse, the value of dietary iodine can be reduced by vegetables from the brassica family, which includes cabbage, brussel sprouts, raw turnip, broccoli, and cauliflower. In circumstances where both large quantities of these foods are eaten and the levels of dietary iodine are marginal, goiter could develop.

Iodine supplementation can be life saving, yet the debate rages on over what is the benefit/risk ratio at what level of supplementation. The issues are complex and not easy to disentangle.

The one thing you can be sure about: we are not getting nearly enough. The problem is that all health professionals hold the delusion that iodine intake is not a problem because it is taken care of by iodized table salt. It's a myth.

For one thing, doctors have been recommending for decades that we all cut down on table salt, Duh!

Secondly, bromine in bread and flame retardants is an antagonist.

> "Fish oil supplementation caused either stabilization or actual regression of tumors.

Thirdly, what you swallow bears no relation to what you absorb. Many people have such a deplorable state of affairs in their gut, they cannot absorb nutrients sufficiently.

Dosage

The traditionalists see the RDA of approximately 150 mcg per day as necessary but adequate. Amounts above 1 mg (1000 mcg) are viewed with alarm and considered potentially toxic. As someone who often takes 30-50 mg in a day, I can tell you that's nonsense.

Doctors are satisfied with iodine levels, if thyroid functions seem normal. I have a problem with that too, which is that thyroid function tests are often clinically worthless; meaning the patient is sick with underactive thyroid, yet they have normal or "acceptable" levels of the thyroid hormones, T4, tri-iodothyranine (T3) and TSH, the thyroid stimulating hormone, which goes up when thyroxin is low.

As in all aspects there is a BIG difference between what doctors consider "enough" and what is optimum. Surely we don't just want enough to stay alive, we want enough to live to the fullest, with vigorous health and mental vibrancy.

I take Lugol's iodine, which has been in clinical use since 1829. It is formulated as follows: 5 g iodine and 10 g potassium iodide mixed with 85 ml distilled water, to make a solution with a total iodine content of 150 mg/mL. Potassium iodide renders the elemental iodine soluble in water. Lugol's is not to be confused with tincture of iodine solutions, which consist of elemental iodine, and iodide salts dissolved in water and alcohol (Lugol's solution contains no alcohol).

I take 5 drops a day (not every day, I'm not a person of habit). This is equivalent to about 30 mgs of iodine.

Organic vs. Inorganic Iodine

Inorganic iodine, as in Lugol's solution, is quite safe. The organic forms (e.g. drugs like Amiodarone and radioactive iodine) are definitely very toxic. Unfortunately, past research has confused the inorganic and organic forms of iodine, resulting in inorganic iodine being inappropriately blamed for problems caused by the organic forms (organic means has one or more molecules of carbon; inorganic does not).

Iodine Loading Test

The Iodine Loading Test was developed for measuring whole body iodine status. It supposes that when the body has enough iodine, it will start excreting any excess. As body iodine increases, a larger percentage of the iodine ingested is excreted. Whole body sufficiency for iodine is arbitrarily defined as 90 per cent or more of the ingested iodine/iodide load of 50 mg being recovered in a 24-hour urine collection. So 90%+ is "normal".

A simpler test is to paint it on your skin. If the yellow stain vanishes in just a few hours, iodine is being absorbed hungrily from the skin, because there is a deficiency. Supplement as above till the yellow stain persists.

Other Nutritional Supplements

Of course you will not need me to tell you that all vitamins, minerals and other nutrients are important and have a place. These are just some key ones I have singled out.

Even so, it is a formidable list. Should you take them all? My answer may surprise you, which is probably not. I know people who take 60-100 capsules and pills daily, as well as rubbing different creams into their skin for absorption.

I haven't the stomach for this sort of thing, which I view with almost as much suspicion as poly-pharmacy. Instead I prefer to take supplements fitfully, as and when I think of them. I also rotate and would never take the whole armory at once. In fact, some nutrients make me feel like throwing up—and that's from a professor of nutrition. So don't take all this too heavily. It's serious but should not be a pain.

My strictly daily supplements include vitamin D, omega-3s and coenzymeQ10 (ubiquinone). I'm convinced that coQ10 and selenium have brought back some of my receding hair. The Mumby's have a strong male pattern baldness gene, yet I seem to have escaped its ravages quite a lot. My two sons in fact are balder than I am. I think it is due to smoking. My father and all his family smoked; so do my sons. I have never smoked and am actually repelled even by the touch of a cigarette.

But nutrition is very important for hair and nail vitality; the two go hand in hand. Even so, I was surprised when my wife spotted new hair growth; not only that, it was dark hair, not silver! Trial and error has led me to believe that coQ10 and selenium are the chief reason for this resurgence.

CoQ10 Update

I'd like to finish up this section with current news on CoenzymeQ10, one of our most powerful and essential anti-agers.

CoQ10 has been around for years. And it's been helpful. But there were major drawbacks to the old type of CoQ10. It was weak and expensive.

The older CoQ10 is called ubiquinon and that was converted into ubiquinol by the body. The trouble was that the body's ability to convert the old style starts to decline after age 45. Traditional CoQ10, the one you find everywhere, is less and less use to an aging individual.

But Japanese researchers discovered a reliable way to skip the conversion process. That means ubiquinol gets into your blood at super high concentrations, with no effort on your body's part.

Al Sears MD is marketing a form of this new CoQ10 which he calls "Accel".

Before this, the dose was 400 mg of the old CoQ10 every 8 hours to keep blood levels high enough. That could add up to a couple of bottles a week and was a very expensive option.

With Accel, most people can get all the anti-aging power with just one caplet a day. That makes the miracle of CoQ10 available to you at a fraction of the cost.

Order your Accel to try through this link: http://bit.ly/coQ10_Accel

8 | The Antioxidants Story

Oxygen Is A Poison!
Despite its status as a necessary life substance for all except a few special organisms, oxygen is a highly toxic mutagenic gas (*Free Radicals In Biology And Medicine*, B Halliwell and J MC Gutteridge, OUP, Oxford 1999, p. 1). We can only survive its presence in our atmosphere because we have important anti-oxidant mechanisms to protect us from its damage.

Initially the earth's atmosphere had less than 1% oxygen. But activity by blue-green algae species billions of years ago gradually increased these levels. For them it was just a waste product of a respiration process that relied on releasing hydrogen from water but for evolution, it was a Godsend.

By 1.3 billion years ago, levels had risen to 1%. Around 500 million years ago, oxygen levels had reached 10%. This was sufficient to switch on the all-important ozone layer, which protects the earth's surface from blazing destructive UV radiation.

From then on, other life forms could evolve.

Oxygen may have reached 35% in the late Carboniferous age, when life was mainly plant-based. The present level of 21% was settled around 5 million years ago. As a result, oxygen is the most prevalent element in the Earth's crust (53%); rock is basically silicon dioxide, with additions.

Definitions
Words like "oxidation" and "anti-oxidants" are used a lot, frequently by people who haven't a clue what they are talking about.

Oxidation has long been taken to mean the addition of an oxygen atom to an existing chemical structure and this is often likened to the process of rusting (rust is iron oxide, formed when iron comes into contact with oxygen in the atmosphere). The trouble is that oxidation in biology is very different.

The broader definition of oxidation is a process in which an electron is grabbed from a grouping. The snatch often takes place violently and essential biological substances can be wrecked beyond repair. Oxidative damage, as it is known, is often held to be one of the main mechanisms of tissue wear and tear during aging.

Taking anti-oxidants is the one way we have of protecting our bodies from the damage caused by this oxidation process. Without anti-oxidants we would die rapidly.

The opposite of oxidation, called hydrogenation, is the addition of hydrogen. By inference, this also means the addition of an electron to an existing chemical grouping.

Respiration

The trouble is, we need oxygen! It is life to our cells. They breathe oxygen and turn it into energy, unlike plants, which get their energy directly from the sun.

About 85-90% of oxygen taken up in advanced animal respiration is consumed by the mitochondria. The essence of metabolic energy production in the body is that food materials are oxidized, by having electrons stripped. This releases the energy to create molecules of ATP (adenosine triphosphate), which is the body's chief energy transport mechanism. The whole process is done in a gradual step-wise fashion, involving the creation of excited forms of iron, from ferrous to ferric-haem cytochrome.

This is a very important physiological detail. It makes iron one of the most destructive oxidative stress elements in our tissues. The removal of excess "hot" iron may be one of the principal mechanisms by which chelation with EDTA reduces or even reverses oxidative age damage.

The whole process is done under the control of a complex enzyme system called the cytochrome oxidase pathway. Cytochrome oxidase in mammals is special in that it works efficiently when there is almost no oxygen present. But xenobiotics and pollution very quickly poison this system, and so render us liable to tissue damage by oxidation.

Reactive Oxygen Species

I don't want to blow you away with obscure language and advanced technical concepts but there are times when you need to understand. I've been told often I make complicated things seem easy to comprehend, so I will try to walk you through this.

We need the fancy words to get the full meaning of the concepts.

The term "free radicals" (hence free-radical damage) was introduced into this oxidation debate. But, strictly speaking, a free radical is simply one capable of existing independently (hence the term "free"); they don't necessarily bite! The radicals we worry about are the ones that are scavenging for electrons; they grab what they want, when they want, even though damage may result.

A better term is reactive oxygen species (ROS). The chief reactive oxidation atom groups (ions) are:

1. Oxygen itself O_2

2. Hydrogen-oxygen paired together, the -OH or hydroxyl ion.

3. The so-called superoxide radical, which is not, in truth, as active or damaging as the basic oxygen radical, despite its name!

4. Ozone is another reactive oxygen species, which is highly destructive to living cells. However, it is little found at sea level, remaining largely in the upper atmosphere, where it shields us from harmful UV radiation. Unfortunately, urban pollution, notably with traffic emissions, in the presence of sunlight, creates dangerous levels of ozone, which we may breathe. It can cause lung damage.

5. Finally, the fifth member of the quintet is the peroxide ion.

Peroxide is one of the most deadly of the bunch and is generated briefly by certain white cells, to kill pathogens before ingesting them. The peroxide is then very rapidly mopped up and removed by the enzyme catalase, to protect healthy tissues.

How critical this is to immunity and how it relates to aging is dramatically seen in full-blown AIDS, where there are few functional white cells, the peroxide control is lost and the body ages alarmingly, often in a matter of just weeks.

So believe me when I say that oxidative damage and anti-oxidant control is of critical importance to successful aging.

Anti-Oxidants

Oxidation stress, leading to tissue damage, has now been implicated in a wide variety of disease complaints, including arthritis, heart disease, cancer, dementias and other degenerative illnesses. Environmental pollution and overburdened lifestyles unquestionably potentiate this aging process.
Smoking and excess alcohol increase oxidative damage also.

> The most sensitive organ to oxidative damage is the brain.

The most sensitive organ to oxidative damage is the brain. This is hardly surprising, since around 25% of the body's metabolic activity occurs in this one organ. This means real changes and loss of cognitive function - "feeling old", lethargy, confusion, and forgetfulness. There are many subtle layers and degrees of this unfortunate process, which we recognize as a loss of zest for life and a failure to think as sharply as we once did.

As we have come to understand the power and significance of oxidative tissue damage, a key process in aging, then substances, which protect us from this occurrence have assumed steadily greater significance in anti-aging science. We call these, not unnaturally, anti-oxidants.

Richard G. Cutler, a research chemist at the Gerontology Research Center, National Institute on Aging, National Institutes of Health from 1976-1995, famously said "The amount of antioxidants that you maintain in your body is directly related to how long you will live".

Different anti-oxidant classes can be listed as follows:

Amino Acids
cysteine, glutathione, methionine, taurine.
Bioflavinoids
anthocyanins (blue-black fruits), citrus bioflavinoids (lemon, orange, grapefruit etc), oligometric proanthocyanidins (OPC) in pycnogenol.
Carotenoids
alpha and beta carotene (red, yellow and orange fruits and vegetables), lycopene (red fruits and vegetables).
Herbs
Gingko, green tea, milk thistle, sage, ashwgandha
Minerals
Copper, zinc, manganese, selenium
Vitamins And Co-Factors
A, B2, C, E and coenzyme Q10, NADH (nicotinamide adenine dinucleotide).
Enzymes
Catalase, glutathione peroxidase, superoxide dismutase
Biochemical Intermediaries
Glutathione

The Ultimate Anti-Ager Of All

The master anti-oxidant, and the original star, is held to be superoxide dismutase (SOD). Compared to vitamin C, this nutrient is 3,500 times stronger. [Colman J. "Life Span-Increasing Effects of Super Oxide Dismutase (SOD)." LEM. Winter 2005/2006.]

In aging studies, researchers discovered mammals that produce the highest levels of SOD have the longest life spans. And according to Cutler, when they genetically engineered fruit flies to have double the amount of this nutrient, the fruit flies lived twice as long. [Cutler RG. "Antioxidants and longevity of mammalian species." Basic Life Sci. 1985;35:15-73 and Cutler RG. "Antioxidants and aging." Am J Clin Nutr. 1991 Jan;53(1 Suppl):373S-9S.

SOD is so vital, production starts when you're in the womb. In another study, genetically engineered mice whose bodies couldn't make their own SOD died in just days from massive free radical damage [Li, et al. "Cardiomyopathy and neonatal lethality in mutant mice lacking manganese superoxide dismutase," Nature Genetics. 1995. 11:376-381].

Without SOD, we would age and die in hours or days from the withering onslaught of oxidative damage. I have likened this in the past to the movie cliché in which an individual is "magically" kept young, but will age and crumble before our very eyes when the magic influence is removed. The movie special effects are not far wrong in showing this happen.

> **Compared to vitamin C, Super Oxide Dismutase is 3,500 times stronger.**

That's how important antioxidants are!

Unfortunately, levels drop off as we age, leading to a build-up of free radicals. [Lishnevskaia VL. "The role of free radical oxidation in aging." Adv Gerontol. 2004;13:52-7]

Moreover, native levels of SOD vary by as much as 50% from person to person, depending on genetic and other factors [Ueda K, et al. "Levels of SOD in Japanese people." Acta Med Okayama. 1978 Dec;(6):393-7]. That may be why some people age quickly and why others live to a ripe old age without any problems.

You should be concerned about how much SOD is in your body. It would be great if we could supplement it but haven't been able to. Till now…

A patent has been passed which claims to have solved the problem of getting SOD absorbed by the oral route, without being destroyed by the digestive process (US Patent 6 04 5809).

The new process wraps SOD in a protective coating, which enables it to pass through your digestive tract without being damaged.

The new patented, absorbable form of SOD is available in Dr. Al Sear's special antioxidant formula RES-3.

You can order it here: http://bit.ly/aHDTaa

Also Rans

A number of other proprietary "anti-oxidant" formulas are on sale. Typically, these include mixtures of vitamin A, beta carotene, C, E, selenium and zinc (so-called ACE formulas, from the primary vitamins). It is advisable to eat plenty of fresh fruit and vegetables, which all contain types of anti-oxidants, as you see from the list above.

Chelation therapy is now known to act primarily as an anti-oxidant process. Elmer Cranton MD, one of the doyen figures of chelation therapy and author of several definitive books, thinks this is mainly by removing "pro-oxidant" ions, such as iron. It may not be all that simple. But the benefits are quite clear.

Just bear in mind that the original concept—that of scouring out blood vessels, rather like Dyno-rod or Roto-router—is rather naive and does not seem to take place (though sometimes Doppler measurements of blood flow can improve dramatically).

Glutathione, The True Miracle

Second only to SOD, glutathione is one of the most powerful anti-oxidants known. It donates millions of electrons and so easily quenches the hunger of scavenging reactive oxygen species. In the late 1990s I started giving glutathione IV, along with EDTA as a chelator, and found startling extra benefits against aging.

Unfortunately, we lose glutathione steadily as we age. It is not known to what degree we age because of this loss.

Glutathione may be the most powerful protective substance in our bodies, because of its other major roles in detox pathways, (see page 77) and stimulating the immune system. I have already pointed out how important the immune system is in preventing aging. Basically, we live as long as our immune system allows us to.

The trouble is that glutathione is lost in the eternal battle against toxins. For every molecule of toxic substance removed, we lose a molecule of glutathione. That makes it very precious.

It is traditionally taught that we can't take glutathione orally; we need the precursors. These are substances that promote the production of glutathione in the body. The main ones are alpha-lipoic acid, N-acetyl cysteine and s-adenosyl methionine (SAMe). They contain lots of sulfur and that's why they are needed: glutathione is a sulfur-rich substance and sulfur is needed in vital phase II detox reactions.

The doses I usually suggest are:

NAC 500 mg daily (any more than that and it becomes an excito-toxin)

Alpha-lipoic acid 200 mgms daily

SAMe 20 mgms daily.

Any other sulfur containing substances are helpful, such as the sulfur amino acids, cysteine and methionine, and even garlic.

Surprise Anti-Oxidant!

A little-known Scottish study looked at the benefits of medicinal plants oils from the herb thyme in regards to brain aging and anti-oxidant protection. I think what they found was significant and a definite "out of the box" anti-ager.

The researchers measured changes in antioxidant enzyme activity and phospholipid fatty acid composition of the aging rat brain and tested whether dietary supplementation with thyme oil or thymol could provide beneficial effects.

Just as with humans, there was a significant decline in superoxide dismutase and glutathione peroxidase activity and the total antioxidant status in the untreated rats with age. This poses a threat of further rapid neurological damage and senility.

Rats fed on thyme oil and thymol maintained significantly higher antioxidant enzyme activities and total antioxidant status than the controls. Moreover important brain fats called phospholipids, which declined with age in control rats, was also significantly higher in rats given either thyme oil or thymol supplement. These results highlight the potential benefit of thyme oil as a dietary antioxidant.

You can inhale thymol or thyme oil or just add lashings of it to cooking (not so good, because of the heat changes).

[Effect of thyme oil and thymol dietary supplementation on the antioxidant status, and fatty acid composition of the ageing rat brain. Aromatic and Medicinal Plant Group, Scottish Agricultural College, Auchincruive, Ayr, UK. Br J Nutr. 2000 Jan;83(1):87-93.]

Attacks On Anti-Oxidants

In February 2007, a shocking attack on antioxidants was launched in an article published by the Journal of the American Medical Association [Mortality in Randomized Trials of Antioxidant Supplements for Primary and Secondary Prevention, JAMA. 2007;297:842-857].

The "study" claimed beta carotene, vitamin A, and vitamin E given singly or combined with other antioxidant supplements "significantly increase mortality". In fact, it showed no such thing and it is typical of the way in which appalling perverted science is published without question by mainstream journals, if it in any way undermines natural health and living.

Even if taking these anti-oxidants really was associated with a higher death rate, the "researchers" completely failed to assess or deal with the possibility that sicker people may be more desperate and more likely to try vitamins and minerals - but are also more likely to die. This would cause a bias showing anti-oxidant takers died quicker. But that's a million miles from saying that anti-oxidants caused the problem!

These hatchet jobs are often done by a "tool" called meta-analysis. That means you pool all the bad studies with those showing good outcomes, mix everything up, fudge all the figures and - hey presto - you cancel out all the good outcomes. This review of 68 studies covered nearly a quarter of a million people and might sound impressive - if you don't know how these stories are faked.

The whole sham study tried to imply that patients were dying of vitamins supplements, when of course they were dying of heart disease, cancer, kidney failure and so on.

Take all the anti-oxidants you can swallow. There are 100,000s of studies showing the benefits. Natural foods are best, colored foods and... chocolate! A BMJ study (December 19, 1998) showed that the more chocolate you ate, the longer you lived. Chocolate is very rich in anti-oxidants: natural unprocessed variety only, I'm afraid!

Polyphenols, Poly What?

Don't worry, this is just a catch-all term that refers to a powerful group of antioxidants from plant foodstuffs. They are the most abundant compounds in the diet, totalling an intake of as high as 1 g/d, which is much higher than that of all other classes of phytochemicals and known dietary antioxidants. For perspective, this is 10 times higher than the intake of vitamin C and 100 times higher that the intakes of vitamin E and carotenoids

Polyphenolic compounds are categorized, according to chemical structure, into flavonols, flavones, flavanones and isoflavones, catechins, anthocyanidins and chalcones.

The collective noun flavonoids, is named for their color (Latin: *flavus*, yellow). Over 4,000 flavonoids have been identified, many of which occur in fruits, vegetables and beverages (tea, coffee, beer, wine and fruit drinks). The flavonoids have aroused considerable interest recently because of their potential beneficial effects on human health - they have been reported to have antiviral, anti-allergic, anti-platelet, anti-inflammatory, anti-tumor and antioxidant activities.

The anthocyanins are deep red to blue-black, depending on pH, and are even more potent anti-oxidants. Generally speaking, the more color, the greater the anti-oxidant activity plants have.

Among the most important members of the polyphenol group are the catechins and epicatcechins. They are the principle reason that green tea has come to have such a reputation as an anti-ager. Chocolate (page 104) is also rich in epicatechins, which is such a powerful antioxidant that professor Normal Greenberg of Harvard has stated it should be classed as a vitamin—meaning "vital amine, essential for life and health"!

That's a new take on chocolate for many!

Green Tea's Powerful Antioxidants

Green tea's antioxidants, called catechins, scavenge for free radicals that can damage DNA and contribute to cancer, blood clots, and speed aging by thickening of the arteries. Grapes and berries, red wine, and dark chocolate also have potent antioxidants.

Because of green tea's minimal processing -- its leaves are withered and steamed, not fermented like black and oolong teas -- green tea's unique catechins, especially epigallocatechin-3-gallate (EGCG), are more concentrated.

Epigallocatechin-3-gallate (EGCG) is the most abundant catechin in green and white tea but does not occur in black tea, due to the fact it is fermented first. EGCG is known to have anti-cancerous properties and can be beneficial in treating brain, prostate, cervical and bladder cancers. EGCG has been shown to bind and inhibit the anti-apoptotic protein Bcl-xl. Apoptosis is good (programmed cell death), so the anti-apoptosis protein is dangerous and EGCG blocks its effect. You may need to read that sentence again, slowly.

A study conducted in Japan that involved nearly 500 Japanese women with breast cancer, found that increased green tea consumption before and after surgery was associated with lower recurrence of the cancers.

Studies in China have shown that the more green tea that participants drank, the less the risk of developing stomach cancer, esophageal cancer, prostate cancer, pancreatic cancer, and colorectal cancer.

Sounds good but EGCG is not readily "available" to the body; in other words, EGCG is not always fully used by the body. So we need to take these wonders with a bit of caution. Nevertheless, I can recommend it wholeheartedly because green tea can do no harm.

Green and white tea, incidentally, have measurable antibiotic properties.

It also seems to be good for the heart and circulation. In a study that involved 500 Japanese men and women, researchers found that drinking at least four cups of green tea every day, may be related to the reduced severity of coronary heart disease among the male participants.

A Dutch study of more than 3,000 men and women found that the more tea consumed, the less severe the clogging of the heart's blood vessels, especially in women.

The trouble with all these studies (including the cancer ones) is that it is difficult to rule out the fact that green tea drinkers may be engaged in other pro-health activities which then turn out to be the real cause of the health benefits, not the tea. Perhaps more of them are vegetarians, for example; or the one I favor, they use less dairy produce, which is a good health preventative in my view.

Milk is poison!

Ashwagandha

This is a powerful anti-oxidant and energy booster. It has a strong claim to be in the anti-aging toolbox. It's full impact has to be fully evaluated. I know some people react badly to it, so ashwagandha may not be a panacea or "elixir of life" by any means.

Try it and see if you can tolerate it OK.

Ashwagandha is a traditional Indian and Ayurvedic herb. It is believed to benefit inflammation, so on that account alone it should help against aging.

But it also described as an adaptogen (resists stress), an immune modulator, an anti-tumor, an anti-microbial, it boosts memory (that too could come from its anti-inflammatory properties).

In a study of mice, Indian researchers found ashwagandha prevented myelosuppression in mice treated with all three immunosuppressive drugs cyclophosphamide, azathioprin, or prednisolone. That is to say, it blocked the destructive effect of chemo, which causes bone marrow to stop producing red and white cells.

Safety is good and side effects are few: however it may cause increased food consumption and unwanted weight gain. It seems to have its energy-boosting effect at least partially by stimulating the thyroid gland. At least one case has been documented of thyroid over-activity (thyrotoxicosis). So don't take it if you have ever had that as a problem.

> A Dutch study of more than 3,000 men and women found that the more tea consumed, the less severe the clogging of the heart's blood vessels, especially in women.

I can't recommend it for hypothyroidism (underperforming thyroid) but I'd try it if I had that condition (wink!)

Usually, marketers suggest 3-6 grams of the dried ashwagandha root a day.

Rhadiola ("golden root") is another "adaptogen" you may come accross. It is generally better tolerated than ashwagandha.

Both Ashwagandha and Rhadiola are found in the product range from Univera, which I highly support.

Ask for the Univera catalogue range by emailing here: admin@informed-wellness.com

Lutein, Zeazanthin and Macular Degeneration

This famous combo are a pair of anti-oxidant carotenoids, known to protect the eyes from macular degeneration. Carotenoids are also polyphenols, natural plant colorants, named for the modern carrot (orange pigments). The original carrot, incidentally, was purple! Dutch growers genetically engineered them to be orange to commemorate their founding father, William of Orange (1533-1584).

Lutein is found in dark green leafy vegetables such as spinach, plus various fruits and corn. Egg yolks are also good sources of lutein. Lutein provides nutritional support to our eyes and skin - the only organs of the body directly exposed to the outside environment.

Source: http://www.luteininfo.com/about

Zeaxanthin belongs to the class of carotenoids known as oxycarotenoids, which contain hydroxyl groups. This makes them more polar than carotenoids, such as beta-carotene and lycopene, which do not contain oxygen. Although lutein and zeaxanthin have identical chemical formulas and are isomers, they are not stereoisomers, as is sometimes believed.

Source: http://www.pdrhealth.com/drug_info/nmdrugprofiles/nutsupdrugs/lut_0164.shtml

ORAC Values, What Do They Mean?

While talking about anti-oxidants, let me address the ORAC values scam that is raging currently. ORAC -- the oxygen radical absorbance capacity -- has meaning only in a test tube yet it has become synonymous with the ranking of berries and consumer products.

Marketers jostle for the pole position by claiming their product has such and such ORAC value and is therefore better than a product with a power score.

It's all a sham!

The ORAC scores apply only to laboratory test tube conditions and were developed and are intended for use by scientists only to quantify the antioxidant potential of such berries used as foods or ingredients.

Armed with such rankings, however, unscientific, unscrupulous marketers proclaim that açaí, for example, is better for you than other berries with lower ORAC scores.

But the ORAC value is a false score that makes no allowance for what happens to a substance after it is swallowed. One of the oldest secrets in nutrition is that what you swallow is not necessarily what the body gets.

You also need to wise up to the fact that the body cannot possibly use any anti-oxidant function running into thousands. Evidence from recent science shows that absorption of ingested polyphenols reaches saturation rapidly, indicating that ability to store such chemicals as antioxidants is limited or non-existent. About 2,500- 3,000 ORAC units is about the most that can be beneficial to the human body.

How The Food Is Prepared

Açaí's exceptional ORAC score is the result of using a specially frozen and vacuum-dried powder -- freeze-dried açaí. No other ORAC scores for berries have come from freeze-dried material that would be comparable to how açaí was prepared.

Freeze-drying is a process usually too expensive for research purposes. Açaí requires special freezing methods rapidly after harvest because the equatorial climate where it grows and its high fat content hasten rancidity.

This special drying preparation accounts for the huge disparities between açaí's high ORAC score and the next berry or fruit in line, whatever it may be (usually given as goji berry but the sea buckthorn peddlers are right in there with their own product).

The reverse of that is that when prepared exactly like other berries and competitive fruits for ORAC, açaí really has quite an ordinary ORAC. Spray-dried açaí powder (heat-exposed juice) or ice-frozen fresh açaí has an ORAC score less than 5,000 units. Rather less than the wild claim of 102,000, which has been stated to be "over ten times higher than the highest ORAC scores for any food…"

Finally, and I think not the least important consideration, you must consider the fact that laboratories are not consistent, one to another. And also, I'm sure, there is a strong tendency to exaggerate values, to keep the customer happy. It's the customers, after all, who pay the salaries!

Just don't be fooled, OK?

Just to finish, here are some reliable and sensible values, published by the US Department of Agriculture.

Top Antioxidant Foods [ORAC* units per 100 grams**]			
Fruits		Vegetables	
Prunes	5770	Kale	1770
Raisins	2830	Spinach	1260
Blueberries	2400	Brussels sprouts	980
Blackberries	2036	Alfalfa sprouts	930
Strawberries	1540	Broccoli florets	890
Raspberries	1220	Beets	840
Plums	949	Red bell peppers	710
Oranges	750	Onions	450
Red grapes	739	Corn	400
Cherries	670	Eggplant	390

* Oxygen Radical Absorbance Capacity

**About 3.5 ounces

Chocolate

This will surprise you: chocolate contains some of the best anti-oxidants known and is a great anti-ager. A study published in the British Medical Journal in December 1998 showed there was a direct relationship between chocolate consumption and a longer life!

You probably thought the opposite: that chocolate made you fat and shortened your life? Actually, chocolate is one of the richest sources of anti-oxidants on this planet! You can get more anti-oxidant power from un-Dutched natural chocolate than from Acai berry.

Now I constantly emphasize that you need to discriminate between healthy chocolate and unhealthy chocolate. But the BMJ study didn't even do that. The more chocolate you consume, even junk sticky bars, the longer you are likely to live, it said!

So, what is it about chocolate that makes it so healthy and what is the difference between "good" and "bad" chocolate? The secret lies in unprocessed dark cocoa solids (what's left after the fat or cocoa butter is squeezed out). That's where the potent anti-oxidants are found.

Unfortunately, the long tradition with chocolate has been to treat it with alkali, the so-called "Dutching" process, and that ruins its health values. Most commercial chocolate (Mars, Cadbury, Hershey's etc) is Dutched and cannot be relied on to the deliver the benefits of true, unprocessed chocolate.

Unfortunately, untreated chocolate solids are very bitter and unpalatable, which means you need to add a sweetener. Sugar, as we know, is a problem, so straight away we run into a paradox: healthy chocolate needs sweetening.

I have designed a special "Doctor's Chocolate" (that's its name). For the sweetener, I used xylitol, a sugar alcohol that is safe for diabetics and has a glycemic score of almost zero. There is next to no fat and my chocolate pieces come in at about 20 calories each; that means it takes 3 of my chocolates for the same calorie score as an apple. Which would you rather eat?

I've been hearing lots of stories from people who find it relieves depression and I'm not at all surprised. Of course, it's just a side effect – hey, we can't help that. You'll just have to get used to smiling more and don't complain about it.

You can find out more about The Doctor's Chocolate by watching videos here:

http://www.doctorkeithschocolate.com

The Science

There has been a flood of scientific papers on chocolate and its health properties. It started with an interest in the health of the people from the island of Kuna in Panama. They have lower blood pressure, less heart disease and fewer strokes than everyone else.

In fact, the death rate from heart disease in these islanders is less than 8% of that in Kuna mainlanders, and cancer incredibly kills only 16% as many islanders as folks on the mainland.

Scientists wanted to know why they were so healthy.

It soon became obvious that the reason was that the islanders drank 4 or 5 cups of chocolate every day – natural healthy chocolate, freshly ground, the kind that I have insisted we use. It was not a genetic factor, because islanders who moved away and stopped drinking the healthy chocolate soon became unhealthy, like the rest of us. They began to get normal rates of heart disease and cancer.

So scientists began to ask what is in chocolate that has such great health benefits? The answer is that it is LOADED with flavonoids.

I expect you would like to know that a small bar of chocolate can contain as many flavonoids as 6 apples, 4 ½ cups of tea or 2 glasses of red wine!

But that's not all. Chocolate contains a remarkable antioxidant polyphenol called epicatechin. It is so good that Dr. Norma Hollenburg, professor of medicine at Harvard Medical School, reckons it ought to be classed as a new vitamin. Why? Simply because, as he says, it protects us from so much harm that it acts exactly like a vitamin. Remember the word vitamin means vital to life and health.

Now the science hasn't stopped just with antioxidants. A lot more good things about chocolate keep us healthy, and keep our hearts beating longer!

Chocolate flavonoids, it has been found, help to relax blood vessels and so lower blood pressure. They also reduce blood platelet stickiness, which helps to prevent clotting – one of the major reasons for heart attacks and strokes. One study showed that a 25 gm bar of good dark chocolate had as much blood thinning effect as 80 mgms of aspirin, used for the same purpose.

Another study showed that chocolate helps the body to process nitric oxide. What does that mean? Nitric oxide is what we need to keep our blood vessels open and functioning. We know now that the chief mechanisms by which we relax our blood vessels and so lower blood pressure. But there is an aside to this; Viagra works by exactly the same mechanism.

Another study showed that chocolate flavonoids were able to alter blood fats or lipids favorably, lowering the dangerous LDL cholesterol and increasing the protective HDL cholesterol. No wonder those Kuna islanders lived so long!

> **Chocolate contains some of the best anti-oxidants known and is a great anti-ager.**

Well, which would you rather do to look after your heart: eat a plate of broccoli and take aspirin every day, with the attendant risk of stomach bleeding, or eat chocolate? I think it's a no-brainer!

Obviously, there are still the party poopers, who live in yesterday's world and have not kept up with the science of today. There's a sort of puritanical streak in this – it tastes good so it's must be bad for you.

Instead of looking at the science, they still quote what Mommy used to tell them: how bad chocolate is. What a shame. If only Mommy hadn't been so ignorant of the facts she could have treated her kids and also eaten chocolate herself. With the appetite suppressant qualities of our chocolate, she needn't have got fat either and so didn't need to fear this awesome food.

We need lashings of anti-oxidants to stay young, so why not chocolate? It's true you can get most of the same benefits from 3- 6 servings of fruit and vegetables per day. But chocolate is tastier, quicker and less hassle.

9 | Hormones, The Good, The Bad, The Ugly

Superhormones Outside The Box

Superhormones are what William Regelson MD, author of The Superhormone Promise, called the "biomarkers of age", that is substances which are a true reflection of the aging process. "As the levels of these hormones decline, so do we, mentally and physically. The loss of these precious superhormones saps us of our energy and vitality, and shaves decades off our lives. By restoring these hormones to their youthful levels, it is possible to restore our youthful zeal and energy, and to strengthen and bolster both our bodies and our minds".

Regelson himself was a superb example of what he preached, busy with writing, travelling and teaching the new gospel of regained sexual vigor and mental vitality well into his 70s. Regelson's "superhormone promise" applies equally to men and women. Nature has given each of us a personal blueprint for age reversal - it is written in our hormones.

However, he was mainly wrong in what he taught. There is no evidence whatsoever that hormones extend life nor that they are causative in the aging process (meaning they could change as a *result* of aging changes, not as the cause of them). This may come as something of a shock to you but I ask you to bear this important point in mind.

Hormones profoundly influence the quality of life, so it's important to understand how they work and supplement those, which are lacking. Quality of life is every bit as important a goal as actual length in years.

One of the first "superhormones" to emerge was DHEA (dihydroepiandrosterone). It precedes testosterone, estrogen, and progesterone. Low levels of DHEA lead to fatigue, depression, loss of vitality and decreased libido. Yet this important substance begins to decline in our bodies from the 20s onwards. By 40, we feel the effects of the loss, and by 80, our DHEA could be as low as 15% of its "youth level".

Another common and important marker is thyroid hormone; if this declines your metabolism slows down markedly.

Of course, estrogen and testosterone are about sexual vigor. More details on this later.

We have melatonin, which works as an anti-oxidant, anti-depressant, and sleep regulator. Melatonin is believed to slow the aging process but interestingly it does not delay the onset of aging, only slowing its progression, so that a longer life may be possible.

Then there is Human Growth Hormone (hGH). In 1990 a major study was published in the prestigious New England Journal of Medicine; author Dr. Daniel Rudman showed that, in real terms, six months of adequate supplementation of hGH was capable of reversing the aging process by as much as 10-20 years; skin wrinkling was reduced significantly, lean muscle mass returned and excess fat melted away, resulting in weight loss even without dieting.

I embraced hGH enthusiastically at first but then the reality set in. Once again, I find myself on the opposite side of the fence to colleagues. Two main reasons:

1. None of the measured effects that Rudman found were true for a person under the age of 70. For anyone below this age, hGH is a waste of money. It does nothing.

2. <u>hGH does not extend life, even by a measurable week.</u> To me, that makes it an almost worthless anti-ager and considering the huge cost involved, I cannot honestly support its prescription.

There are so many approaches to anti-aging that do extend life—often very significantly. To me these are the way to go, not costly prescription medicines that may have hidden dangers.

Growth Hormone: Who Needs It?

In this context "growth" hormone is a misleading term. It does not cause significant growth once the bone end plates have fused – in other words from late teens onwards. In this younger age group, growth hormone is used to overcome dwarfism and is very successful. It has been quipped that today it would be very difficult to find a cast of munchkins for a remake of "The Wizard of Oz"!

I have already mentioned the now-famous study published in the prestigious *New England Journal of Medicine* in May 1990. Dr Daniel Rudman and his team at the Medical College of Wisconsin, Milwaukee tested the benefits of human growth hormone injections (hGH) on volunteers in their 70s and 80s. The result was quite clear: six months of injections reversed the aging process by 10-15 years in patients who received the hGH, measured in terms of bone density, lean muscle mass, loss of the belly fat, improved cardiovascular risk profile, more energy, and an overall feeling of well being. In the control group that didn't receive hGH, the normal aging process continued.

Since then, the results have been echoed many times. A review of the literature by the Society of Endocrinology posted on their website states that, overall, at least 80% of patients given growth hormone replacements demonstrate a significant improvement, especially in fat distribution, body composition and parameters reflecting well-being and quality of life.

So what's the problem? Why don't we all take it?

The answer is there may not be a problem. But skeptics are cautious: in theory at least, growth hormone can trigger a spurt of growth in a tumor, though there is no evidence, hGH actually causes tumors in adults. It can make you ugly: some degree of bone growth will take place and this emerges as thickening of the brows, chin, wrists, and other appendages, which may not look very attractive. Also, hGH will cause the major organs to grow and a large heart and kidneys may not be a good thing at all.

There is the point I made: that Rudman's study concerned men in their 70s and 80s. It does not infer that people in a younger age group will also gain back 10-15 years. In fact, there is no real support for taking hGH on a permanent basis, unless you are very old and decrepit and this is, so to speak, the "last ditch".

What You Can Do

If you are considering hGH, the first step is to find out if there is a problem. Serum hGH levels can be measured but this is technically very difficult, since it is released by the pituitary gland only at night, in short spurts. It is better to rely on testing another substance in the blood, which mimics the activity of hGH and that is called insulin-like growth factor-1 (IGF-1). Most laboratories today can measure this easily. Dr James Frackleton, one of the founding members of the American College for the Advancement of Medicine (www.acam.org) gives a simple formula, which he says is useful to work out what your personal IGF-1 level (usually reported in nanograms per mL) should be:

$$\text{Calendar age} = 115 - (\text{IGF level})/4$$

Just to make this clear, say the IGF-1 level was 260 ng/mL and substituting in the equation:

$$\text{Calendar age} = 115 - 260/4 = 115 - 65 = 50 \text{ years old.}$$

If this person was fifty years old, the IGF-1 level is just about right. If he or she was 40 years old, it would be too low. On the other hand, if he or she were 67 years old, this individual would be doing quite well!

If you are concerned and would like to consider injections of hGH, then you must discuss it with a knowledgeable medical practitioner who has specialized in this field. Do not be put off by the inevitable bluster or platitudes of doctors who are not up to date on this. But if you do go through with it, do not take hGH for more than one year total in maximum (for life), until more is known. I might suggest, say, 3 months one year, 3 months a year later and then 6 months five to ten years after that.

However, if you have weighed the risks versus your desires and decided you do not want to administer hGH until we know more (which is sensible), or you are still not old enough to be in the major league for hGH, there is still a great deal you can do.

Firstly, we know that hGH always declines with obesity. So get some pounds off if you haven't already done so. Also, exercise unquestionably helps. Start taking walks, running, dancing, whatever you fancy, but get on the move frequently (see Chapter 14).

This is a lifestyle commitment. You must make major changes if you want to live long and live well. Remember hGH is only a tiny part of the story. All good health advice is valid. Good nutrition provides the vital building blocks for prolonging zestful life. It makes no sense when doctors, as we have seen, prescribe hGH for their patients, yet have not implemented these three simple basics first. You will feel tons better in life by eating less, eating right, stacking up your antioxidants, exercising more and taking proper vitamin and mineral supplements.

Follow the advice I give elsewhere in this book.

Secretogogues

Unfortunately, hGH has spawned a whole industry on the Internet and pay television, offering compounds which are claimed to stimulate the secretion of hGH. All quote the Rudman study for spurious credibility. But it does not apply; the Milwaukee study examined only the effects of injected hGH, nothing else.

The buzz term is "secretogogue", a hybrid word which sounds convincing but means nothing. "Hormone precursor" is another favourite phrase. The claims are large, since there is a fortune to be made by those who can gull the public. Just remember you are being sold herbs, amino acids and minerals—not hGH!

However, there are things you can take which have been shown to possibly enhance hGH levels and these are worth considering.

Top of the list was gamma hydroxybutyrate (GHB). One Japanese study showed that it increased hGH by 16-fold. Unfortunately, GHB is also the notorious "date-rape drug" and no-one is now likely to be able to obtain it for anti-aging purposes. But a derivative compound, gamma amino butyric acid (GABA) is readily available and offers some value as an hGH stimulant. GABA is a neurotransmitter. It is also a relaxant and will make you drowsy, so take GABA only at night. Perhaps its effects come from creating better REM sleep, which we have already stated will increase hGH levels anyway.

One of the main purposes of GABA within the body is to preserve and regulate muscle tone, which makes it a popular ingredient in supplements designed for bodybuilders. However, the muscles of the face also benefit from the effects of GABA, explaining why GABA is a prominent ingredient in many anti-aging treatments such as supplements, serums and anti-wrinkle creams.

Take 500-1000 mg GABA in powder or capsule form at night.

Other amino acids, which may work as hGH-releasers are ornithine, lysine, arginine and glutamine. Ornithine definitely helps release hGH. It can be synthesized in the body from arginine, which therefore makes more sense as a nutritional supplement. The additional benefits are that arginine helps prevent the memory deterioration notoriously associated with aging and it is a good relaxant for blood vessels. The latter means arginine is good for blood pressure and also male sexual performance.

Lysine boosts the effects of arginine. Take 500 mgms of each.

Remember you will also need the amino acids cysteine and methionine to supply sulphur, so that your regenerated skin will be smooth and elastic! Sulphur also helps the joints and stops them being so creaky. Finally, take tyrosine along with co-factor iodine, to help boost the thyroid (**page 95**). It's no good for a car to have a new paint job if the engine is still running sluggishly!

Proper medical supervision by a knowledgeable physician is preferred in supplementing these compounds, since arginine and lysine may release insulin as well as growth hormone. We now know that raised insulin levels can be damaging and definitely shortens life, so beware. Generally when hGH levels are rising, insulin levels are falling. IGF-1 will also increase and as its name suggests it is a growth and repair trigger, which will restore tissues, but it also mimics insulin. If you can't get skilled help, 500 mgms of each amino is almost universally tolerated. You can adjust the amounts of each until you feel best and your IGF-1 is where is should be.

Learn more here: www.endocrinology.org/SFE/gh.htm

Men's Stuff

The male essence you might say is testosterone. But remember that male bodies also carry significant amounts of estrogen. Since we don't really understand why it's there, the boffins have tended to say it's unimportant. But when I was a medical student, they said that about the thymus gland, which we now know is one of the most important organs in the body and regulates T-cells (T for thymus)!

Similarly, women have traces of testosterone. Amongst other things, it drives their libido, so both ways it's pretty important to us guys.

Testosterone gets a bad press. It's supposed to make us harsh, aggressive and insensitive. I'm sure it does in excess. But lack of it leads to torpor, depression and negativity. That's not having a "feminine side"; that's sickness.

The fact is we men need testosterone, not the least because it protects us from heart disease. For years, the stupid myth was that since women have fewer heart attacks, testosterone causes cardiovascular disease. Probably it raises blood pressure, because it makes men energetic and goal driven; that's stress, right?

Just another example of scientific bovine excrement! One day, somebody got to wondering if this myth is actually true. He studied the testosterone levels of men lying in intensive care units, having suffered stroke or a myocardial infarction (heart attack). What was found was that men with cardiovascular problems had far lower levels of testosterone than average, not higher. It emerged that testosterone actually protects from heart disease; totally the opposite of what "science" had said. Incidentally, that's true also for women. When their testosterone levels drop later in life, they eventually assume a similar risk to males.

Testosterone generates strength and stamina. It regulates youthful protein synthesis, lowers cholesterol, reduces blood sugar levels and fortifies bone density. Dr Eugene Shippen MD, author of

The Testosterone Syndrome, points out that this is not just a "sex hormone". Testosterone is a whole body hormone.

So we need that stuff. Enough to feel good, to protect our arteries and live longer, but not enough to make us road freaks and intolerant bullies! Otherwise, lacking it, we slide into a male equivalent of the menopause, which has been dubbed the andropause. Characteristically the man begins to lose energy and drive; depression, demotivation, and loss of libido follow. Physical decay is soon part of the picture.

It's bad news for the wife or partner. Men are hard to live with even when they feel good about themselves; it's ten times worse when their virility deserts them!

Note there is a phenomenon called the "midlife crisis", which is rather different from the hormonal andropause. I have a whole section later in this chapter, to help you understand the important difference.

> **Testosterone generates strength and stamina. It regulates youthful protein synthesis, lowers cholesterol, reduces blood sugar levels and fortifies bone density.**

Testosterone Supplements

Supplementing testosterone has been around for a surprisingly long time. Pioneer work by Dr Tiberius Reiter and his followers in the 1950s showed dramatic results. As a result, there were queues of men outside his door and scientific orthodoxy, typically, ignored the new breakthrough in healing. The know-alls went on decrying the idea of such a thing as the andropause (the majority still does). When the drug industry finally got into the act, the result was a disaster.

True-to-form, a synthetic patentable analogue of natural testosterone, called methyl testosterone, was brought onto the market. It worked okay but caused a lot of cancers. As a result, testosterone supplementation was discredited and even today ignorant reactionaries cite this tale with dire prognostications (absurdly, methyl testosterone is still licensed in the US by the FDA but safe natural testosterone preparations are attacked).

The fact is there are safe ways to supplement testosterone these days; Restandol or testosterone undecoanate is one. Capsules, patches and implants are available, each with relative merits and problems. If you are hesitant, take only the natural testosterone molecule and avoid any modified patented compounds. Good anti-aging clinics will supply a gel formulated from pure natural testosterone, just as nature makes it. I used to prescribe a 3% cream with great effect. 5% should be used with care.

CAUTION Aromataze

The picture isn't quite as simple as it sounds. This is due to the fact that some testosterone is converted into an unwanted estrogen form, by an enzyme called aromataze. *A 60-year old man has, on average, more estrogen then a 60-year old woman.*

It is this "male estrogen" or xeno-estrogen (measured as sex hormone binding globulin or SHBG) which leads to prostatic enlargement and NOT testosterone itself, as you may have been led to believe. Male estrogen also adds to the risk of heart disease.

Dosing is therefore not a matter for self-treatment. Blood tests are required to learn the existing levels of SHBG. If it's high, this tricks the pituitary and interferes with the secretion of LH (luteinising hormone), which then scores low. LH is meant to stimulate the testes to secrete testosterone. If LH is high and testosterone low, the regulation pathway is probably OK but the testes are not responding to the signal.

We also need to block the aromataze pathway, to prevent the conversion into male xeno-estrogen, which is otherwise bad news. Failure to grasp the importance of this side path is the chief reason for ineffective and mismanaged male hormone supplementation. Even if you are not contemplating testosterone supplements, this build up of male estrogen can put you in danger, through heart disease and through prostate cancer. At the very least, you will tend to feminize, as older men do.

Known antagonists of aromataze are saw palmetto and zinc. If you are supplementing testosterone, you MUST take at least 300 mgm of saw palmetto and 50 mgm of zinc daily. Saw palmetto may also block metabolism of testosterone to androstenedione, another potent androgen that has been implicated in prostate disease.

Also good news is that plants in the crucifer family (cabbage, kale, broccoli and brussel sprouts) contain large amounts of an estrogen antagonist called indole-3-carbinol, I3C for short. This has been shown to be very helpful against women's estrogen dependent cancers, such as breast and cervical cancers. We men can benefit from the same breakthrough. Eat plenty from this group.

Chrysin (passionflower), available as capsules or cream also has a definite beneficial effect in this context. Avena sativa (oats) is also said by some to increase free testosterone.

If the SHBG cannot be brought down to safe levels, it may be wise to consider a drug called Arimidex (anastrozole). It is prescribed to breast cancer patients, to eliminate the estrogen problem. For a male using it in this way, the correct dose is no more than 0.5 mgm 2-3 times a week. Obviously, this is a prescription-only matter.

Arimidex is NOT used routinely with testosterone supplements.

Finally, see the section on *Peuraria mirifica*, later in this chapter.

Vitamin K and prostate

This is much more important than most doctors recognize. The EPIC study at Heidelberg (it really was an epic: 11,000 men over an average of 8.6 years) showed conclusively that vitamin K gives critical protection against prostate cancer. It showed that K1, the plant derivative, was not helpful but K2, menaquinone as its known, did the job well. K2 lasts far longer in the body.

Moreover, K2 is known to protect our arteries and be helpful in preventing osteoporosis.

The current recommended intake of vitamin K in Japan is 55 mcg for women and 65 mcg per day for men. In the US and Canada it is 120 mcg per day for men and 90 mcg per day for women. These figures are disastrously low (as usual) and need to be at least tripled. I repeat K1 will just NOT do the job.

Take 300 mcg daily, minimum if you are a man (or woman) over 55.

CAUTION: Do not use external applications of testosterone if you have physical contact with children: there is a case on record of a male child going into premature puberty through contact with testosterone cream on his father's body. Do not use testosterone if you have a raised PSA or known prostate cancer.

Which Brings Us To Prostate Health

As a medical student, I heard male patients being told "If you get a cancer, choose the prostate". This tumor is a very slow killer and survival for 20 or more years is not unusual, even without treatment. Many men die of something else, without ever realizing they had an invader, munching away slowly!

Nevertheless, that's a pretty stupid reason to accept it when cancer of the prostate is among the most preventable of all malignancies. Its appearance is all but confined to later years in life and the cause, apart from the general causes of malignancy (DNA decay, nutritional factors and chemical carcinogens), is the steady build up of male estrogen. This leads first to benign prostatic hypertrophy (BPH) and sometimes then on to cancerous growth.

Prostate specific antigen (PSA) is the usual screening test but hardly a gold standard. It may be negative in the presence of cancer and may be positive when there is none. Nevertheless, to not have regular PSA checks from middle age onwards is walking blind. Checks are mandatory as a preliminary to supplementing either growth hormone or testosterone on an anti-aging program.

Where there is clear enlargement of the gland and a problem SHBG level, it is vital to raise free testosterone (as opposed to bound testosterone) as a protection and at the same time block the conversion to estrogen. Saw palmetto and zinc are given, as above. While restoring testosterone levels to a normal healthy level (25- 40 pg/mL) does not cause prostate cancer, it has been suggested that it may induce faster growth in an existing tumor. However, a study from Santa Barbara in California showed that testosterone actually killed the tumor cells. That's more in keeping with the physiology outlined here.

Tossing Away The Risk!

Men could reduce their risk of developing prostate cancer through regular masturbation, researchers suggest [BBC News Site, 16 July, 2003, 23:11].

They say cancer-causing chemicals could build up in the prostate if men do not ejaculate regularly.

And they say sexual intercourse may not have the same protective effect because of the possibility of contracting a sexually transmitted infection, which could increase men's cancer risk.

Australian researchers questioned over 1,000 men who had developed prostate cancer and 1,250 men who had not developed prostate cancer, about their sexual habits.

They found those who had ejaculated the most between the ages of 20 and 50 were the least likely to develop the cancer. The protective effect was greatest while the men were in their 20s.

Men who ejaculated more than five times a week were a third less likely to develop prostate cancer later in life.

Fluid emission could be the key.

Women's Stuff

A woman fights aging in a way which men do not. There is something deeply psychologically important to a woman in her looks and the alteration in physical beauty that accompanies the transition into middle age is often disturbing and humiliating for her. Yet celebrity figures like Elizabeth Taylor, Raquel Welch and Joan Collins have shown that traditional beliefs in when a woman looks her age have to be revised considerably.

> **A woman's life is controlled by hormones in a way which is much more pronounced than the male.**

The battle against aging really begins before the menopause. And as I advise all patients, anti-aging is really only about good general health. To the degree you eat the right foods, take adequate nutritional supplements, minimize stress, exercise regularly and form good sleep habits, to that degree you are engaged in anti-aging. But there is one extra dimension for a woman – hormones!

A woman's life is controlled by hormones in a way which is much more pronounced than the male. Imbalances can wreak havoc with a woman's psyche, persona, and physical well-being. Traditionally, this has been ignored, or written off as mere "womanish" things; scorn or impatience has more often been handed out than sympathy and effective care. Until recently, science has largely failed the fair sex. Self-prescribing and the search for "alternatives" is a sure sign that the mainstream is out of tune with the problem.

We understand things a little better now. Hormone replacement therapy (HRT), though seen as a menace by some, has transformed many women's lives from hell into something more normal. It is my certain belief that we will come to understand more and more about this aspect of health physiology and that the benefits will increase as we do so. It is an especial interest for many scientists and doctors that we try to find as many natural regulatory methods as possible.

Age is not a prison or a penance (even though it has been viewed that way in the past).

We come back to HRT.
With the advance of years, women suffer a decline in their vital sex hormones, estrogen and progesterone. After giving due attention to establishing and maintaining good general health and vigor, it makes sense to restore levels of these hormones to more youthful levels. Estrogen-like activity in particular is important, in that it protects against loss of bone density and heart disease. Diminished secretion of estrogen may result in a degree of masculinization, which is unacceptable. More importantly, it may mean the woman is assuming a male risk profile of heart attacks and stroke.

The trouble is that estrogen is perceived as dangerous, owing to the role it plays in stimulating certain tumors. This is only half-scientific; you will readily see that women in their teens and twenties, with floods of these "dangerous" hormones in their blood, do not have a higher incidence of cancer of the cervix or breast.

However, we know for sure that after the Women's Health Initiative Prempro study, published in 2002, breast cancer rates in the US fell by a dramatic 15%. This is almost certainly because women, millions of women, stopped taking Prempro, a synthetic menopausal hormone replacement therapy. The WHI study, a large clinical trial looking at Prempro, made by Wyeth, found that women taking the estrogen-containing drug had higher breast cancer rates and more heart attacks, strokes and blood clots. Within six months, the drug's sales had fallen by 50 percent.

Following this (the very next year), the incidence of the all breast cancer types, started to downturn and dropped by 7 percent in 2003, or about 14,000 cases, according to a recent report by the National Cancer Institute. This is the first time that breast cancer rates have fallen significantly since 1945. Up till now, the rates had climbed steadily (despite all the propaganda that we were supposed to be "winning" the Cancer War!)

The biggest decrease overall was seen in women ages 50 to 69. That is the group most likely to have been taking menopausal hormones. Of course Wyeth dispute that their synthetic drug could have any such effect as causing breast cancer (they would, wouldn't they?)

The use of estrogen to treat menopause took off in 1966, when a doctor, Robert Wilson, wrote the best-selling book "Feminine Forever" and flew across the country promoting it. He insisted that estrogen could keep women young, healthy and attractive.

He was wrong; he made his $millions. And women died.

But now there is a really good alternative; almost a wonder drug in its own right.

The Miracle Herbal Hormone
Pueraria mirifica (also known as *Kwao Krua* or *Butea Superba*) is a plant found in Thailand and Myanmar. The region where this plant is grown is remarkable for its low rate of breast cancer and impressive longevity. Mirifica means "miracle maker" and it seems as if we have a miracle herb on our hands. You could call this new product HRT with a spin = herbal rejuvenation therapy or herbal remedy from Thailand!

Beware what you read about this plant. Here are the scientific facts.

The PM plant tuber contains phytestrogens such as miroestrol, deoxymiroestrol, which are found only in Pueraria mirifica. **Miroestrol is thousands of times more potent than soy or red clover isoflavones**. The Thai government is supporting the commercial production of this product and backing research.

The UK journal *Nature* was the first to publish consolidated information on PM in 1960. The Thai Ambassador to the Court of St. James supplied the root sample to The National Research Laboratories in London. There a team led by Dr. James C. Cain built on research published as early as 1940. Their conclusion was that PM was at least a hundred times as rich in estrogenic activity as red clover. 40 years later, it has been calculated to be around 3,000 times the estrogenic activity of soy isoflavones. Yet, as an adaptogen, it does not exhibit a rise in blood or urine estrogen levels.

PM appears to work by blocking estrogen receptors, yet has no direct estrogen activity itself, which is why it is so incredibly safe and protective against breast cancer.

Men (60 years and older) should maybe take PM too. I have already explained that some male aging effects are due to the accumulation of "male estrogen". But don't suppose it will take the place of good diet, exercise, cutting down on alcohol and losing plenty of belly fat (which is where male estrogen "lives").

Side effect or bonus?
You may end up with enlarged breasts! This is almost a side effect but P*ueraria mirifica* is now being promoted commercially for breast enhancement. You can buy it on eBay. Someone is even producing a chewing gum called B2Up (Bust-up Gum). Predictably, I suppose, it was a big hit in Japan, where girls long for (supposed) Western-style melons on their chest.

The first acknowledged human study on breast enhancement was done in 1999 by Professors Kuramoshi (Japanese) and Yuthana (Thai). They tested [certified] PM species on 50 Japanese women, between 20 and 49 years old, with daily doses of 100 mg to 600 mgs / day, following our current recommended schedule of the 8th day from the start of the monthly menstrual cycle to the 21st day.

Tests carried out by Thailand's Chulalongkorn University found *Pueraria mirifica* gel was able to enhance breast size by up to 80%. Further tests carried out in England found that the plant had a beneficial effect on the skin, and hair, as well as the breasts.

[To date there have been no valid structured tests demonstrating the efficacy of breast creams containing PM].

Authenticity
Your biggest challenge with this amazing herbal supplement is getting authentic supplies. There is very little available and it is closely controlled and certified by the Thai government.

Butea Superba and 13 species of Pueraria growing in Thailand are all called Kwao Krua. Butea (a completely different species) is Red Kwao Krua and Pueraria are called White Kwao Krua. PM is one of the white species family members. Black Kwao Krua is a totally different species and has little to no valid research. Unlike White Kwao Krua, Black and Red Kwao Krua grow throughout most of South East Asia. PM also grows in a small mountainous area of Burma, extending from Thailand's northern border. Otherwise, it's only (99%) grown in Thailand.

Basically, over 90% of stuff on the market is fake. Creams said to contain PM may actually contain one of the other 12 Pueraria species, or even a combination of a number of species. One, sold in Malaysia, has evidence of containing synthetic hormonal precursors. Despite the fact that they do work, there have been a number of negative reports from users. Synthetic hormonal precursors will do that.

Start your search for authentic PM here:

Smithnat pharmaceuticals (http://www.smithnat.com/miracle_herb.html)

The two US suppliers I stand by are as follows:
- Solgar (www.Solgar.com, where you can download literature)
- LongevityPlus (www.LongevityPlus.com)

You can hear me interview Dr. Sandy Schwartz, CEO of Smith Natural Pharmaceuticals, the main producer of clinical grade Pueraria, at this page:

http://www.AskDoctorKeith.com/pueraria_mirifica.htm

Pregnenolone: The Mother Hormone

You will sometimes hear DHEA described as the "mother hormone". The term would be better applied to pregnenolone, which is the basic precursor, or starting raw material, for the production of ALL the human steroid hormones, including DHEA, progesterone, estrogen, testosterone, cortisol, and aldosterone. But pregnenolone is not itself steroid hormone.

Pregnenolone has been studied extensively since the 1940's, when it was used both experimentally and medically. Pregnenolone was phased out of medical use; yet ironically pregnenolone is radically safer and more versatile than the specific steroid hormones, which replaced it! Pregnenolone is safe even at 1 gram (1000mg) dosages, a claim no steroid hormone can make (20 mgms or more of prednisolone, one of the main synthetic prescribed steroids, would be dangerous long-term).

One of the most important actions of pregnenolone is to counter damage caused by the cortisol. Cortisol is helpful in modest amounts, but toxic at higher levels. Amongst other things, it damages brain function and this can lead to blunting of normal memory. Blocking this process may be one of the main reasons for the known memory-enhancing effect of pregnenolone. It also improved the mood and efficiency of factory workers, which may also be due to benefiting brain function, as well as enhancing mood.

Other actions of pregnenolone include limiting allergic reactions and reducing inflammatory processes, such as arthritis. By now you should be clear on the powerful anti-aging benefits of quenching inflammation.

Pregnenolone also improves energy levels by protecting our energy-producing mitochondria from environmental toxins.

The body's own production of pregnenolone is reduced with aging, stress, depression, hypothyroidism and toxin exposure. The work of Ray Peat PhD has shown that pregnenolone may be a general "anti-stress" metabolite. However this may not always be present in our bodies at optimal levels, precisely because it may be used up in producing all the steroid hormones, not leaving enough to fulfill its stress buffer role. Hence the need for supplementation.

Pregnenolone is generally safe and effective at doses of 50 mgm to 200 mgm per day. If you are self-dosing, judge it from your mood and energy levels. On no account use pregnenolone instead of medically prescribed steroids, without telling your doctor what you are doing.

DHEA

In a sense, DHEA started the anti-aging movement. One of the pioneer books was *DHEA Breakthrough* by Dr. Stephen Cherniske. There have been many claims that DHEA is the secret to preventing certain diseases and more importantly as the "fountain of youth."

> **An 80-year-old person has 10% to 20% of the DHEA that a 20-year-old has.**

DHEA can be taken as a dietary supplement and you can also increase your DHEA levels with strenuous exercise on a regular basis. However, taking a DHEA supplement is a good way to ensure that your level increase and remain consistent.

An 80-year-old person has 10% to 20% of the DHEA that a 20-year-old has. That's because the amount of DHEA in the body decreases dramatically as a person ages. DHEA is believed to significantly reverse the aging process when taken as directed.

Natural DHEA decreases are related to the development of Alzheimer's, multiple sclerosis, diabetes, arthritis, Parkinson's disease, cancer, obesity, heart disease, atherosclerosis, and depression.

DHEA It is the most abundant hormone in the body and it is the most dominant steroid hormone. Humans produce more DHEA than any other species.

However DHEA levels significantly decline with age, and this decline has been correlated to varying degrees with many of the complications associated with aging, such as cardiovascular disease and high cholesterol levels, insulin resistance and diabetes, obesity, and neurodegeneration. In humans, DHEA has been reported to reduce body fat, alleviate angina, and reduce LDL ("bad") cholesterol, and it has also been used to treat cancer, multiple sclerosis, coronary artery disease, lupus, Alzheimer's, HIV/AIDS, depression, PMS symptoms, and osteoporosis.

It has antiproliferative effects on some human cancer cell lines [Steroids. 2004 Feb;69(2):137-44. Antioxidant effects of dehydroepiandrosterone and 7alpha-hydroxy-dehydroepiandrosterone in the rat colon, intestine and liver. Pelissier MA, Trap C, Malewiak MI, Morfin R.].

In animals, DHEA has been reported to decrease body fat and have beneficial effects in rodent models of diabetes, lupus, anemia, atherosclerosis, and breast, colon, lung, and skin cancer. It also improves memory performance and has immunostimulating and antiglucocorticoid properties.

DHEA is also good for sexual health and is considered an excellent general tonic to keep sex hormone levels thereby increasing ones libido. For these reasons, DHEA has been termed "fountain of youth" [Bioorg Chem. 2002 Aug;30(4):233-48. Ergosteroids VII: perchloric acid-induced transformations of 7-oxygenated steroids and their bio-analytical applications--a liquid chromatographic-mass spectrometric study. Marwah A, Marwah P, Lardy H].

DOSE: the usual dose recommended clinically is 25-50 mg for a man. However a woman taking such levels would likely get spots and greasy skin. I found that 15 mg was about the maximum a woman could take, without running into this inconvenient side effect.

DHEA results occur gradually building over time so don't expect instant results. Patience is key to enjoying the benefits. The anti-aging properties of DHEA are also gradual but then so is the process of aging.

Unwanted Effects

DHEA is not without its problems. For example, it converts to both estrogen and testosterone and hence subsequently unwanted "male estrogen".

[Mol Cell Endocrinol. 2003 May 30;203(1-2):13-23. Evidence that dehydroepiandrosterone, DHEA, directly inhibits GnRH gene expression in GT1-7 hypothalamic neurons. Cui H, Lin SY, Belsham DD.].

In animal studies, high doses of DHEA increase liver weight and the risk of liver cancer.

[Drug Metab Dispos. 2004 Mar;32(3):305-13. Stereo- and regioselectivity account for the diversity of dehydroepiandrosterone (DHEA) metabolites produced by liver microsomal cytochromes P450. Miller KK, Cai J, Ripp SL, Pierce WM Jr, Rushmore TH, Prough RA.].

7-Keto DHEA

A better idea may be to take a metabolite of DHEA: 7-Keto was originally developed to avoid the unwanted hormone-like effects of DHEA.

Tests in animals show 7-KETO is a thermogenic (fat-burning) compound. Thermogenesis is the production of heat from the body's metabolism: the higher the degree of thermogenesis, the more fuel is burned. Your body's metabolic rate will increase, using up ingested or stored calories at a higher rate. Great for weight loss.

7- KETO can lower cholesterol, improve memory and leads to a decrease in unhealthy triglycerides in the liver. It has a beneficial effect on immune system function and according to one Czech study can mitigate the harmful effects of cortisol.

An even better study, presented in April of 2004 and reported from the Minnesota Applied Research Center and the Geriatric Research Education and Clinical Center in Minneapolis found that 7-KETO supplementation improved immune function in elderly men and women. This randomized, double-blind, placebo-controlled study involved 22 women and 20 men over the age of 65. They were given 100 mg of 7-KETO twice daily, or a placebo, for four weeks. Researchers noted that patients in the 7-KETO group had a significant increase in immune helper cells and a significant decrease in immune suppressor cells. There is also an increase in neutrophils - white blood cells that are the first to respond to infection.

DOSE: 100-200 mg daily seems about right.

Blood And Saliva Tests

Hormone levels are best detected with a comprehensive blood test that measures your full range of hormones. However saliva testing can give important guidance on levels and can be arranged by post, which is convenient for most patients.

Individual hormones should not be considered in isolation, as they interact and depend on each other to a surprising degree. Some basic suggested test panels include:

For women:
- Estrogens (estradiol, estrone and estriol)
- Progesterone
- DHEA
- Thyroid stimulating hormone (TSH)
- Cortisol
- Free testosterone (women should have traces of testosterone, which are important to libido and sexual health).

For men:
- Free and total testosterone
- Estradiol
- DHEA
- Thyroid Stimulating Hormone
- Sex-hormone binding globulin (SHBG)
- Cortisol
- Prostate specific antigen (PSA) (in case testosterone replacement is needed)

You will need to work with a skilled, licensed physician to correct what comes up. But persist in demanding help. You'll be amazed at the transformation in mental wellbeing that can come about when a low thyroid or estrogen dominance is properly corrected.

Obviously, in the anti-aging arena, we are talking mainly about deficiencies. But that is by no means always the case.

Cortisol, in any case, we want down, not supplementing to increase it. It's the number one PRO-aging hormone, as I have explained elsewhere.

Get saliva testing for hormones at this laboratory: http://www.diagnostechs.com

10 | Heart And Vascular Health

Cut Your Risk of Sudden Death by 92%. It's official!!

One of the Roman Emperors, I think it was Julius Caesar, when asked how he would choose to die, said "Unexpectedly." It's a neat point. None of us want to linger miserably; so dropping dead in the street when you least expect it has a certain appeal.

But not if it's twenty years before your time, surely?

The disease that usually produces sudden death is a myocardial infarction (MI) or, to the layman, a "coronary thrombosis". More exactly it is a sudden loss of the heart's contracting rhythm called fibrillation, as a result of some serious damage, usually (but not necessarily) a clotting episode in a coronary artery. By "sudden" we mean there was no prior warning; the patient was unaware of any health problems.

Obviously, this is more likely to happen as you get older. But even if you are not in your 5th, 6th or 7th decade or older, don't get smug. One of the shocking developments of the 20th century was seeing young people, apparently fit and in their prime, dropping dead due to a heart attack. We lost some great people that way: Richard Beckinsale (British actor), Florence Ballard (The Supremes), Cass Elliot (Mamas and Papas), Maggie Sam (American blues guitarist), Big Moe (rapper), Mario Lanza (operative singer) and many more, still in their 30s.

What a waste!

Of course as the years go by, you are more and more likely to die of all causes and sudden death, whether a heart attack or catastrophic stroke, also increases as a risk. Note that these are both, basically, diseases of the arterial system. Until recently, this was the West's number one killer (it's been overtaken by cancer but only because cancer is badly managed and doctors insist on turning it into a death sentence by stupid and destructive treatments).

You should always keep in mind that arterial disease is very dangerous, often very insidious (hidden) and always very widespread throughout all tissues. The cardiac surgeon who tells you that just replacing a few inches of corroded artery near the heart will fix you up good is a shocking fraud!

What he or she really means is that they get richer; you're just that bit further on the road to death; nothing has really been solved. Bad arteries in the heart invariably mean bad arteries to the kidneys, liver, brain and other vital tissues. You have rotten plumbing.

That includes blood supply to the brain. Probably nothing causes senility (dementia) more than poor nutritional supply to the brain, caused by aging and inadequate arterial supply.

As well as senility, stroke is an ever-present risk too. This too produces many deaths, often quick and tragic, if not in minutes then certainly within hours of the disaster. Even if the patient survives but can no longer talk to his or her loved ones, that's a pretty sad version of "survival", you'll agree.

A New Disease

The joke is that this carnage is entirely avoidable; the rotten-artery disease hardly even existed a century ago. That alone should tell you it's largely environmental; despite what you hear: genetic factors are almost irrelevant (eating habits are "inherited" and they are what kills the individual).

> **Arterial disease is very dangerous, often very insidious and always very widespread throughout all tissues.**

The layman has heard of "hardening of the arteries"; the medical word is arteriosclerosis, which means just the same thing. You may also encounter the words atheroma and "plaque". These refer to plates of hardened foamy grease stuck to the walls of an artery, which narrow it and spoil its smooth anti-clotting properties. Thus not only is blood flow imperiled by narrower pipes but a fatal clotting process is much more likely, once this condition is established.

Want to opt out? You can and should.

Once again, this is an entirely remedial condition. Though mainstream medicine believes, with a zeal bordering on fanaticism, that what you've got you are stuck with, the truth is you can repair and mend your blood vessels to an astonishing degree. Countless studies and trials have proved this; though of course the evidence is always swept under the carpet by an industry obsessed with granting power to the drug companies, rather that attaining health for its patients.

Well, a new study (Oct 22, 2007) puts paid to all the crooked flummery.

It's from Sweden, opportunely enough. I ran an international clinic there for a time, first in Gothenberg and then Stockholm, commuting madly back and forth from the UK each month. It was a lovely time and if you ever get chance to go see Stockholm and its beautiful 24,000 island archipelago, I encourage you to do so.

The Swedes were always the let-it-hang-out nation of Europe. Into nudity and sexual freedom long before anyone else, so no-one could ever accuse this nation of wanting to cover up anything!

A team under Dr Agneta Akesson (Karolinska Institute, Stockholm, Sweden) looked at the benefit of a combination of several healthy lifestyle behaviors and found that most myocardial infarctions

(MIs) in post-menopausal women could be prevented by consuming a healthy diet, being physically active, not smoking, and maintaining a healthy weight. Don't be disappointed this was only for women: in fact, although heart disease is more prevalent in men, it's a little-known fact that sudden death is commoner in women.

The value of this intelligent study was that it showed clearly the benefits of combining different health strategies, something scientists are often loath to do. They study individual factors and never seem to care that when you combine different parameters the results come out very different sometimes.

> **If you combine all these strategies you can get a massive 92% reduction in the risk of a myocardial infarction and, by inference, sudden death!**

Whereas we all know that stopping smoking or exercise or eating healthily or being the right weight is good and will produce some health benefit, usually around 10-30% different, *if you combine all these strategies you can get a massive 92% reduction in the risk of a myocardial infarction and, by inference, sudden death!*

"Our study shows the great effect you get from each of these and by combining them," said Dr. Akesson. "It's quite a simple health message, and you can do them by yourself."

This was no small-scale study either. The Swedish group assessed behavioral dietary patterns among the 24,444 postmenopausal women, who were already participating in the population-based prospective Swedish Mammography Cohort and who were free of diagnosed cancer, cardiovascular disease, and diabetes mellitus at baseline (September 15, 1997).

Akesson and co. identified four major dietary patterns: healthy (vegetables, fruits, and legumes); Western/Swedish (red meat, poultry, rice, pasta, eggs, fried potatoes); alcohol; and sweets (sweet baked goods, candy, chocolate). Those who consumed moderate amounts of alcohol (5 g or more a day; equivalent to a glass of wine every other day) were categorized as low risk. No upper limit for alcohol consumption was defined; because few women consumed high amounts of alcohol (less than 0.3% reported drinking more than 45 g/day).

Those who did best ate an almost fourfold higher weekly consumption of vegetables and fruits, a threefold higher consumption of legumes, and a 70% higher consumption of fish compared with those who did worst.

If you ate well and kept alcohol within bounds, you would have a significant 57% reduction in MI.

But the 5% of the study population who ate healthily, drank alcohol only in moderation or not at all, kept their weight down and exercised regularly had a MASSIVE 92% decrease in risk of MI, compared with women who broke all the rules.

The population-attributable risk in the study population, in which only 5% of the women fulfilled the criteria for the comprehensive low-risk behavior, was 77%, "which suggests that more than three of four of the coronary events could potentially be averted if all women would change their behavior to the low-risk profile," the researchers explain.

I've been teaching all these elements for years but this is the first time that scientists have taken the trouble to study all the elements in combination. Other studies, for example, have looked at MIs and diet, but many assessed only dietary behavior and did not include alcohol intake or the combination of these with other healthy lifestyle approaches.

A similar study in the New England Journal of Medicine looking at the Nurses' Health Study did find a similar reduction in MI, although this study used the somewhat outmoded body-mass index as a measure of obesity, rather than the better waist/hip ratio adopted in the Swedish study.

All these new revelations support something I've been saying for 15 years: the average life expectancy is rising slowly, but I believe that buried in the overall figures is a group of people who have far healthier and longer lives, because they really take care of themselves. If you separated these individuals from the obese, lazy couch slobs, their success statistics would stand out clearly. Studies that do so, like this one, are rare.

Of course there will be those who say "This only applies to women," or "This applies only in Sweden," or "This isn't valid, it was not a double-blind controlled trial." Really, I've heard these dumb arguments many times. The other tactic is not to try and discredit good science like this but just to ignore it and continue the ride on with the surgical gravy train, as if nothing had happened.

Dr. Akesson concluded that, although randomized trials would be best to establish causality between both diet/lifestyle and coronary heart disease risk, such randomized trials are difficult to perform for multiple risk factors. As a result, the combined low-risk behavior would probably never be able to be tested in properly. Therefore, prevention should build on best available information.

How wise.

[Akesson A, Weismayer C, Newby PK, et al. Combined effect of low-risk dietary and lifestyle behaviors in primary prevention of myocardial infarction in women. Arch Intern Med. 2007;167:2122-2127]

Blood Pressure is a Killer

There is a long-standing medical aphorism that "a man is as old as his arteries". This applies equally to women, of course. One of the major degenerative changes associated with aging, at least in the civilized world, is the gradually process of hardening and narrowing of the arteries we call arteriosclerosis or "atheroma" (sometimes atherosclerosis). Clogging lumps of thickened matter in the artery wall we call "plaques"; this is not the same as dental plaque but then, as you will learn here, there are important similarities.

The bad news with hardening of the arteries due to atheroma is that it raises blood pressure (hypertension), because the pipe conducting fluid is narrower. This makes the heart work harder and is the cause of increased prevalence of heart attack and premature death. Hypertension also increases the risk of stroke, which is the next major killer, after heart attacks.

Clogging of the arteries to the legs (resulting in gangrene) and arterial "blow outs" (aneurysms) are other unpleasant manifestations of this condition. In fact arterial degenerative disease accounts for one-half of all the deaths, which take place in the Western world.

But the effects are much more widespread than this. Silting up of the arteries takes place all over the body and one of the many results of this is reduced nutrient supply to the tissues. This can be particularly critical for the brain, which has a high rate of metabolism (page 95).

Poor blood flow means not enough oxygen and brain food; therefore thinking becomes slowed and confused. Over the years this can degenerate into senility and dementia. Arteriosclerosis is the main recognized origin of dementia conditions in the elderly. But the kidneys, liver and other organs suffer reduced blood flow too and so cannot perform effectively in detoxing the body.

In short, the saying that the state of your arteries determines the effective age of your tissues is quite appropriate. You must look after your arteries for a long and healthy life.

The Cholesterol Myth

That's right, you read it correct. The cholesterol story is a myth. It's there only to sell dangerous statin drugs. Saturated fat is fine. It's synthetic fats that cause the problem. Transfats are notorious. But even the once-healthy polyunsaturated fats (PUFAs) are dangerous, if they are not natural (as in margarine). See, essential fatty acids (EFAs), such as omega-3s, are also polyunsaturates. So loading the system with fake PUFAs actually displaced the good stuff and makes matter worse, not better.

The joke is that we NEED cholesterol; it forms the basis of hormones like testosterone and estrogen, the very substances we need as we age. Lack of adequate cholesterol is deadly for aging. It will kill you.

So when I see people boasting their cholesterol level is only 140 mg/dl or so, I feel worried for them. They are pretending good health and will pay for it with an early demise. It's yesterday's science coming to the surface once more.

You've probably heard of "good" and "bad" cholesterol. Those are high-density lipoproteins and low-density lipoproteins, respectively. The more HDL you have in proportion to LDL, the better; HDL is protective, not dangerous.

But also dangerous are our serum triglycerides. The joke is that triglycerides, like cholesterol, are necessary to life. So whenever possible (that is, for about 8 hours after a meal), the liver takes up dietary cholesterol and triglycerides from bloodstream. During times when dietary lipids are not available, the liver produces cholesterol and triglycerides itself.

Elevated cholesterol and triglyceride levels can be caused by several factors, including heredity, poor diet, obesity, sedentary lifestyle, age, and gender (premenopausal women have lower cholesterol levels than men). Several medical conditions, including diabetes, hypothyroidism (low thyroid,) liver disease, AND chronic renal (kidney) failure, can also increase cholesterol.

Get them in the range they need to be. But NOT, please not, by taking drugs. Drugs do not solve the situation at all. These abnormalities are solved by correct diet and adequate healthful supplements.

Just remember: abnormal blood fats are not the CAUSE of anything; they are the result of health issues. In the same way that the engine oil warning light is not the cause of mechanical problems, but rather the result.

Dating Your Arteries

There is a method, which can date the "age" of your blood vessels and then compare this to your actual age. It actually measures functional change in your arteries, which of course, precedes the notorious structural changes which are so familiar and widely studied (atheroma). The sophisticated electronic sensor system does this by measuring the shape of the pulse wave that travels down your arteries.

The test is simple: you wear a clip sensor on one finger for a few minutes and the machine does the rest. It looks at pressure, blood flow, velocity and profile throughout the whole pulse wave. What should be there is a wave pattern with multiple aspects to the wave, or at any rate at least two "bumps". That means your arteries are bouncing back, the second "bump' shows how nice and elastic (ideal) your arteries are (think of a rubber ball bouncing).

As we age this second "bump" disappears, showing that the arteries are no longer elastic but more like rigid metal pipes. I have avoided terms like "dichrotic" (double or bi-polar) and hope you follow this simplified rendering!

This reliable test goes beyond EKG and other tests, which rely on electrical activity. Not very good because when electrical activity vanishes, you die in seconds. In other words any change is very late and the consequences quite serious. Measuring functional elasticity makes more sense, easier to do, fast and can be done by anyone with a few hours training. No special licensing or skills required.

Therefore, inevitably, it's very inexpensive, typically starting around $100! That's why you won't hear about it from cardiologists or the rest of the dollar-hounds. The machine is called a digital pulse analyzer (DPA).

I found a short video showing you a bit more of this type of device here:

http://www.youtube.com/watch?v=rhH4_zhuWWI

The DPA provides information on arterial wall stiffness and determines the biological age of arteries in less than 3 minutes. It has FDA 510(k) clearance, which means you can claim the test on insurance.

Dr. Keith special insights

Myocardial infarction, stroke and artery disease were unknown until the start of the 20th century. People ate lashing of saturated fat: butter, curds, cream and cheese. Yet the modern plague of heart attacks and stroke did not even exist. You'll search for it in vain in medical texts of the day.

Then along came margarine: fake, plastic, unnatural fats. Within a few years we had atherosclerosis and heart disease!

The attack on saturated fats is nonsense and unscientific. Eskimos have traditionally eaten a diet LOADED with fats: about 40% by some accounts. Yet Eskimos do not have heart attacks. If anything their problem is bleeding, not blood clots! (Eskimos consume a great deal of fish oils, containing EPA and DHA, powerful omega-3s that inhibit inflammation and blood clotting).

Don't worry about dietary fat or your cholesterol levels. Being told to avoid cholesterol foods is stupid. Your body makes far more cholesterol than you could ever swallow.

Eggs contain a lot of cholesterol and people have been warned off eggs for 2 generations. The result: an epidemic of senile macular degeneration of the eyes. Eggs contain two powerful substances, which feed the eyes: lutein and zeaxanthanine. Miss out on your eggs and you are hurting your eyes a lot (other sources, incidentally, include: kale, spinach, turnip greens, collard greens, romaine lettuce, broccoli, zucchini, corn, garden peas and Brussels sprouts).

Dozens of clinical research studies and pharmaceutical trials have already been completed utilizing this technology, involving more than 2,500 subjects, and resulting in more than 30 scientific articles published in peer-reviewed medical journals.

Good news for me, by the way. I'm 64 but my arteries are actually 38 years old! Good news for my wife too since, as I keep telling you, blood flow is everywhere in the body!

The Inflammation Connection

Modern thinking about arterial disease is in terms of what have been nicknamed "stealth pathogens", meaning hidden micro-organisms within the body. These are by nature chronic infections and the reason is that the organism manages to disguise itself from the immune system, rather like the US "stealth fighter" makes itself invisible to radar.

The most notorious culprit for this is *Chlamydia pneumoniae* (related to the Chlamydia which causes venereal infections) but others include viruses of the herpes group (again related to but not the same as the genital herpes virus), cytomegalovirus (CMV) and Epstein-Barr.

Interestingly, all these organisms tend to produce a muted, grumbling, difficult-to-clear disease, even when they have been spotted by antibody radar, so it is in their nature to progress to chronic hidden infections. There will probably be more of these pathogens to emerge as time and study progresses.

This is all part of a new view of aging which can be called the inflammatory basis of aging (see Chapter 3).

When a stealth pathogen invades our blood vessels, it slips into the lining of the arteries and then puts up its invisible defense. Sometimes antibodies are a clue, but even when present, our immune system seems unable to clear the invader adequately. The problem is such that by the time we reach the age of 70 over 90% of the population have positive antibodies to *Chlamydia pneumoniae*, the chief gothic villain in this drama. Antibiotics are not the simple, attractive answer that they may seem, since the antibiotic cannot penetrate into the infectious pockets where the organism hides.

However, an inflammatory process does take place and it is now thought to be this process, which is what really damages the artery walls. First streaks appear in the blood vessel lining, this then acts as a seat to attract deposits of fats. Low density lipoproteins, or "bad cholesterol", in particular passes into the wall of the artery and there it is oxidized to dangerous rancid forms.

This in turn is gobbled up by macrophages, which become glutted and are termed "foam cells". Clumps of these start off the plaque, which was what scientists formerly thought was the actual cause of the problem. So fatty plaque is not the real problem but the body's solution to the problem! Fibrous growth to wall off the site of inflammation completes the picture, further hiding the real culprit, and inevitably the arteries grow stiffer and narrower.

Now we can understand why LDL cholesterol is bad for us and why levels of unoxidized cholesterol never was the real problem. It also reinforces the urgent importance of us all taking daily large doses of antioxidants; apart from general protection against free radical destruction, antioxidants prevent the LDL turning into the oxidized form, which is what causes the progression to foam cells. Pristine unoxidized LDL does not initiate this cascade of changes.

Plaques Are Not Where It Starts

But there is yet another astonishing change in our view of things arterial. Previously it was thought that a fatal heart attack or stroke was caused by the artery becoming progressively narrower and narrower, until one day the pinch was too much and the cells of the heart or brain tissue being supplied were suddenly cut off from oxygen and died dramatically.

We now know this is rare. Only about 15% of heart attacks take place where the artery is badly scarred and thickened by the inflammatory process. Recent careful post-mortem examinations have observed that the majority of heart attacks and strokes come from tiny undetectable plaques, which rupture into the blood stream and cause a sudden clotting or thrombosis episode.

This, at last, offers an insight into the mystery of why many fit slim people, who take supplements and work out, even so die suddenly of a heart attack.

It also makes it obvious that angiograms, with all their attendant risks, are pretty worthless since they do not show up the truly dangerous plaques, only the ones which nature has already dealt with. For the same reason, bypass surgery is rarely justified and does not give any better results than passive treatment, long-term. It's not attacking the real problem and as such is mere flim flam dressed up as medical show biz!

What You Can Do

By all means have your doctor obtain an ordinary cardiac risk blood profile. This features especially total cholesterol, HDL, which is protective cholesterol and LDL, which is bad cholesterol. You also need triglycerides. There is no doubt statistically that raised triglycerides put you in the high risk category, though by now you will be aware that this does not mean triglycerides are necessarily to blame. Triglycerides are only the marker, not the problem.

You also need to take into account how much exercise you get and whether your waist measurement exceeds 40 inches. If both factors are negative, this add greatly to the risk.

One of the best markers for risk of heart disease, not altered by the new theory, is plasma homocysteine. This is not done routinely and you will need to ask for the test. It should be below 8; above 10 is poor; above 12 is definitely dangerous. But the good news is that homocysteine can be brought down by administering just three vitamins: B6, B12 and folic acid. If yours is high, you will need help from the doctor. B12 needs to be injected and folic acid 5 mgms a day is a prescription-only medicine. Add 50 mgms of B6 daily.

Sad to say the ordinary general practitioner would need this spelled out.

If you have unhealthy levels of any of the blood fats it would be best to work on correcting them. As I said already, you do not need statin drugs or other synthetic substances. You need, as always, good nutrition, good lifestyle, stress-free conditions, plenty of exercise and adequate antioxidants and other supplements.

> **Artery damage can be reduced by many other factors discussed in this book.**

Remember that artery damage can be reduced by many other factors discussed in this book. For instance, testosterone has been described by one of the world's leading nutritional doctors as a "heart hormone", so good are its protective effects against arteriosclerosis. It was once thought that testosterone aggravated heart disease (men suffer more than women). It is now known that almost all male sufferers of arteriosclerosis and heart attack have seriously low levels of testosterone.

Reduce Inflammation at all Costs

The key survival/longevity factor is to reduce inflammation at all costs. Fortunately, our knowledge is expanding rapidly in this direction. Scientists have learned of a progression of chemicals called prostaglandins, which in turn are derived from essential fatty acids. Surprise! - there are good prostaglandins and bad ones.

The bad sort trigger inflammation but we can't eliminate them. Instead we must make sure that they are opposed by plenty of the good sort. Unfortunately, the typical western diet is low on the essential fatty acids that lead to the best protective prostaglandins, which are made from omega-3s. This is made worse by the fact that fast food is loaded with omega-6s, from corn oil and similar food enhancers, which effectively squeeze the omega-3s even more and make them seem even more deficient.

In other words we need much more omega-3s. You will often hear the Eskimos cited as having a diet rich in omega-3s, which is why they did not, traditionally, get heart attacks or stroke (no longer true now they eat our food). Incidentally, they ate a diet very rich in fats, which tends to put paid to the old myth that the fat you eat is what kills you. Fat is essential in our diet, to absorb vitamins A,D and E, and to obtain EFAs. *But it must be the right sort of fat.*

Omega-3s come mainly from seafood though for those of you who don't like seafood, flax seed (linseed) contains plenty. If you buy commercial sources, make sure they are fresh. Nothing turns fat rancid faster than exposure to air. Rancid fat is deadly in our bodies.

Incidentally, the very best source of omega-3s will surprise you and that's grass-fed beef. Real grass-fed beef, mind, the beasts that have lived all their life grazing, not just turned loose in a field a few weeks before slaughter!

Heart Savers

We have dealt with arterial degenerative disease in some detail, since it is important to everyone who wants to live long and live well. Here we can consider some important alternative treatments, when heart attacks or angina have already become the problem.

First of all, let's be clear about what we mean by these terms. Angina is a constrictive pain in the chest, provoked by exertion. It is the body's signal that the blood supply to the heart is inadequate, due to poor arteries. A "heart attack" occurs when the blood supply to heart muscle is suddenly shut off, by a clot or obstruction. The layman's term was "coronary thrombosis"; doctor's don't use this label but you may hear them referring to a "myocardial infarction", which translates as death of heart muscle due to interrupted blood supply, that's all!

The muscle may simply stop beating or, more commonly, it goes into an irregular pattern (ventricular fibrillation), which no longer works like a pump. This is usually fatal, and death takes place within a very short time, unless someone can apply immediate cardio-pulmonary resuscitation (CPR). It's something everyone should learn and one day you may save a life with this simple skill.

However very many people survive their first heart attack. Experts tell us that if you live through the first 60 minutes after such an attack, you have a good chance of making it. The question then is: What to do? You or your loved one has had a warning that things are wrong, dangerously wrong, and you must act, to prevent further episodes, any one of which could be the last.

Specialists will recommend drugs and/or by-pass surgery or other operative procedures. It is important that you realize that **not one of these medical or surgical treatments attempts to solve the cause of the problem, only the result of the problem.**

The cause is decades of self-neglect and poor lifestyle. Understand that and you can still pull it around and live another forty years or more! Some people have gone on to run a marathon after their first heart attack. You don't need to aim for that but your immediate target is to get healthy. That means three key things:

- Diet change (nutrition and weight loss)
- Exercise and activity
- Reduce stress

These alone will save you. But you may be offered by-pass surgery (grafts), stents (artificial tubes) or angioplasty (scraping out the obstruction, like drain cleaning). Surgeons will try to panic you into action and tell you, like salesmen, that if you are quick, they might just save you. You need, if at all possible, to remain calm and even at these moments of stress.

Hopefully, you will have already read this section and learned this one important fact: apart from one unusual variation, a surgical operation will not help you live longer. *Major hospital studies have shown repeatedly that by-pass surgery is a waste of time, in terms of survival.*

Couple this with the fact that the operations are dangerous: 1 in 10 patients have a further heart attack actually during bypass surgery and more than 1 in 50 die (2.5% mortality). One study at the Montreal Heart Institute in Quebec showed that 20% more surgical patients died than in the group, which was left alone. Also a degree of brain damage is an almost universal unwanted after-effect, which can cause significant personality change (due to hours on an artificial heart-lung machine).

If you can keep your wits while you are being subjected to scare tactics, you might wonder if there is any alternative. Actually, there are two major treatments, both safe and effective, we would like to tell you about. Both have been around since the 1950s and have proven their worth.

Everyone should be made aware of these options but they are kept from the public by a jealous and money-motivated profession. One is called **external counter-pulsation** and the other is known widely as **chelation**, though I prefer the term **intravenous antioxidant therapy,** for reasons I will explain.

External Counter Pulsation

The name might seem a little intimidating but the principle is simplicity itself. The patients wears five blood pressure cuffs, one on each calf, one on each thigh and one on the buttocks (hence "EXTERNAL") – a computer arranges that the moment the heart relaxes between beats, these cuffs are thumped in such a way as to send blood backwards and so into the heart muscle (hence "COUNTER PULSATION"). It is really like having two hearts: one which beats properly and then a second heart beat, slipped in while the real muscle organ is relaxing.

The double blood supply to the heart is terrific and nourishes it when being starved has been the problem. Some three dozen or so 1-hour treatments are needed in all. Patients who have undergone ECP, as it is called, report feeling many extra benefits, such as increased activity, improved quality of life, better vision, and a return of sexuality. Medication can be reduced or even eliminated altogether. A single treatment has positive effects, which can last for a week or more but after a full course, bypass surgery or angioplasty can be deferred for many months, years or even indefinitely.

ECP is a simple out-patient procedure and requires a minimum of time off work. No injections or invasive tubes are required.

Intravenous Chelation Therapy

In the 1950s, doctors treating industrial lead poisoning using intravenous EDTA (ethylene diamine tetra acetic acid) noticed something unexpected: the patients also seemed to recover from blood pressure, angina and heart incapacity; fitness and walking performance improved.

The results were so good that doctors began at once to treat arteriosclerosis with repeated EDTA infusions. The new method was given rave write ups in the medical journals of the day. Chelation, as this technique is called, became the new way of treating heart disease, safe, economical and, above all, highly effective.

Unfortunately, within a few years, a new specialty hit the limelight and that was open-heart surgery. With the event of efficient heart-lung machines that enabled completely emptying the heart, glamorous new surgical possibilities opened up, such as heart transplants and artery by-pass grafts; the media-hype for this hatchet surgery went wild and chelation seemed to be forgotten. Cardio-thoracic surgeons everywhere wanted it buried because it was cheap competition for their very expensive (and largely worthless) antics.

Now, several decades later there is considerable controversy: chelation is carried on much as before but by a small band of doctors who fit the definition of holistic, while the multi-billion dollar heart surgery industry savages them with claims that chelation doesn't work and is a fraud. The original research is forgotten and politics has come into play (one professor even changed his position and said that his clinical trial which showed that chelation was effective really didn't show that at all).

Yet bypass surgery, as I have said, has not proven its efficacy. In fact almost all research shows that it is a waste of time. But that won't stop the juggernaut of greed and fabulous incomes trampling on the true facts.

The Chelation Facts

Chelation saves lives, with a fraction of the pain and risk involved in major open-heart surgery. But benefits are measured not only in terms of heart disease; patients who have had chelation report feeling better, more zestful, increased sexual performance, better eyesight and even improvements in dementia and Parkinson's disease. Wrinkles and age spots are reduced dramatically. Even bone density can improve – good news for those with osteoporosis.

Part of the controversy has been that chelation doctors cannot adequately explain the success of the therapy. It was originally thought to be due to removing calcium from the artery walls; this is now no longer held to be the case. What is known is that EDTA is a very powerful antioxidant (it is used as such as a food additive) and thus can reverse some of the effects of aging, by quenching free radicals.

But perhaps, after all, the real reason is the original reason: that EDTA is great at removing metal poisons from our bodies. Metal poisoning is one of the most destructive biological hazards we face in our environment today (section 14).

Like ECP, chelation is a simple, inexpensive, out-patient procedure. Each treatment takes about 3 hours and a course of 30-50 would usually be called for, depending on the severity of the patient's condition. That's still a cost of less than $5,000, compared to $50,000 and upwards for bypass surgery.

It is important to remember that neither surgical intervention or these simpler procedures will help you at all, unless you take seriously the three lifestyle heart savers listed above.

Vitamin K2

Vitamin K2 is important. The K stands for "koagulation" (it was discovered in Denmark, where they can't spell!) and vitamin K2 is essential for the process of clotting. Coumadin (warfarin, Jantoven, Marevan, and Waran) has the opposite effect, by blocking vitamin K2, and is a real disaster.

Coumadin causes calcification of the coronary arteries, which we now hold is the number one predictor of heart attack! Blood vessel calcification is frequently found in patients with osteoporosis, atherosclerosis, and chronic kidney disease, leading to high morbidity and mortality rates. That's why you'll hear me say over and over "Who needs calcium supplements?"

Well, K2 is found to clinically reverse coronary artery calcification. Do not wait for high calcium counts on hi speed coronary CAT scans to start prevention. K2 will help remove calcium and restore the natural elasticity of blood vessels.

K2 really is the ideal antagonist to Coumadin. That means you need to be careful. You need plenty of vitamin K2 but should make sure that this is not speeding up your clotting time and increasing the risk of an adverse clot in the heart or brain. If clotting time does decrease markedly, your doctor will want to reduce the dose. But better is lots of omega-3s, the ideal way to safely balance K2 and keep the blood "thin".

Recently there have been two other developments to the K2 story, which have made it remarkably compelling. K2 helps prevents bone loss (osteoporosis) and also fights weight gain and obesity.

Ideally you need about 500 mcg a day. If you already have significant calcification of the coronary arteries, try for about 10 mg. It's somewhat complicated by the fact that the "dose" is not equivalent to the active ingredient but I'm offering guidelines on what quantities to look for in a supplement. Unfortunately, K2 is expensive (about $10,000 a kilo I'm told), so decent supplements will reflect this.

Vitamin D3. Now Here's a Surprise!

Vitamin D excess causes calcium overload. I'm not even arguing with that. I can only say the vitamin D excess is very rare indeed! What's far more important is that experimental data show that vitamin D3 inhibits the calcification of arteries, at reasonable serum levels *and* it benefits chronic kidney disease. Low levels of vitamin D3 have been shown to lead to increase of calcification, so there is a paradoxical effect or as we say in science "biphasic" action: too much is bad, too little is bad!

You need 1500-2000 units daily but check your calcium levels and keep them within bounds. I take 4,000 units. The best check, by the way, is accurate bone densitometry. Serum levels vary little even when there is a huge excess or deficiency, because the heart would stop if this was allowed to happen. But if there is a deficiency, the body will rob the bones to prop up blood levels of calcium.

Notice I said accurate bone densitometry; the machine at our local Eisenhower (Kaiser Permanente, I think) is really very bad. It conveniently over-estimates bone loss and so sells more Fosamax and other junk drugs for treating the "problem" it has created.

[Curr Opin Lipidol. 2007 Feb;18(1):41-6. Links Vitamin D and vascular calcification. Zittermann A, Schleithoff SS, Koerfer R. Department of Cardiothoracic Surgery, Northrhine Westfalia Heart Center, Ruhr University Bochum, Bad Oeynhausen, Germany. azittermann@hdz-nrw.de]

Arterial Scurvy

Just to complete the picture, Thomas Levy MD has pointed out the clinical dangers of low vitamin C status.

One area where resistance to good nutrition seems to be evaporating is vitamin C's cardio-protective effect. Even as little as 100 mg/day has a measurable effect. Some studies showed that improvements max out at this intake.

However, the First National Health and Nutrition Examination Study (NHANES I) epidemiologic follow-up study found that 300 mgms a day (including supplements) reduced the risk of death from cardiovascular diseases by 42% in men and 25% in women.

A 2003 study published in the Journal of the American College of Cardiology followed up more than 85,000 women over 16 years, also suggest that higher vitamin C intakes may be cardio-protective. Levels of around 360 mg/day were associated with a 27-28% reduction in coronary heart disease (CHD) risk.

Vitamin C and Hypertension

The protective effects of vitamin C go beyond heart benefits. Several studies have demonstrated a blood pressure lowering effect of vitamin C supplementation. One recent study of individuals with high blood pressure found that a daily supplement of 500 mg of vitamin C resulted in an average drop in systolic blood pressure of 9% after 4 weeks. It should be noted that those participants who were taking antihypertensive medication continued taking it throughout the 4-week study.

> **The risk of stroke in those who consumed vegetables 6-7 days of the week was 54% lower than in those who consumed vegetables 0-2 days of the week.**

Vitamin C protects against stroke too. A Japanese study, following residents of a rural community for over 20 years, showed that those with the highest serum ascorbate levels were 29% less likely to get a stroke than those with the lowest ascorbate levels. This was a valuable study, because it measured actual serum levels, not just the dietary and supplement intake of vitamin C.

Additionally, the risk of stroke in those who consumed vegetables 6-7 days of the week was 54% lower than in those who consumed vegetables 0-2 days of the week. In this population, serum levels of vitamin C were highly correlated with fruit and vegetable intakes. Unfortunately, this makes it difficult to separate the effects of vitamin C on stroke risk from the effects of other components of fruits and vegetables. But it does emphasize the benefits of a diet rich in fruits and vegetables!

Reducing Clotting Tendency

Just as important as the condition of your arteries is the chemical cascade that leads to blood clotting. How likely is your blood to clot, given a risky situation? If a small plaque ruptures yet the clotting process does not take place, there may be no problem. That is how anticoagulants work and why aspirin is protective – it thins the blood. Aspirin reduces inflammation too, which also ought to help, and maybe anti-inflammatory drugs will have a place.

Blood which flows thickly is more likely to clot and we call this property the "viscosity" of the blood. Bags of anti-oxidants and plenty of omega-3 fats is the way to reduce your blood viscosity and so minimize the chance of unwanted clotting.

This also has bearing on what happens in your body after you may have had a clot. Viscosity and clotting factors dictate how quickly the problem may be cleaned up (clot busting) by the natural process of healing.

Special tests can detect the presence of friendly clot-busting chemicals in the blood and also the baddies, what the scientists call "adhesion molecules", the ones which trigger those sudden deadly clots caused by ruptured plaque. Although the body can protect itself to a degree, as Dr Peter Libby, Professor of Medicine at Harvard and co-author of Heart Disease, a classic textbook of cardiology points out in the May 2002 edition of SCIENTIFIC AMERICAN, *"inflamed plaques release chemicals that impede the innate clot-busting machinery".*

Most important is the measure of blood levels of a substance called fibrinogen. This is one of the most important inflammatory markers, as I already mentioned in Chapter 3. Ask your doctor or knowledgeable holistic practitioner to carry out this test. This is the actual substance from which clots are produced and if high it clearly poses more risk.

And yet again, I have to emphasize how important it is to get down levels of inflammation in your body—at all costs.

Why do You Need to Know?
Because you can favorably influence levels of fibrinogen in your blood, it tends to rise as we get older and is made worse by obesity, smoking, diabetes, and the presence of LDL. But fibrinogen is reduced by exercise, raising HDL and – good news – alcohol in moderation.

Vitamin E has long been held to reduce blood clotability. But a word of caution: it needs to be the *right kind of vitamin E.* Alpha tocopherol, which is common and likely to be prescribed by your doctor (since at least one drug company makes it), is wrong when taken alone. Tests show that the whole range of the vitamin E family is required: beta and gamma tocopherol plus tocotrienols. Just alpha tocopherol on its own may make things worse. This is the important information behind the repeated claims that vitamin E doesn't work: it's not real vitamin E!

Formulations of the other tocopherols in combination are now commercially available. Look for them.

Niacin (100- 1000 daily) and Vitamin C (2 grammes daily) can also modestly reduce the clotting substances.

11 | Brain Savers

The Brain and Aging

No organ is more critical than our brain, which means the wear and tear of aging will show up first in thought function; we begin to get slower in our movement and manners, easily muddled, more forgetful and eventually a little silly.

Shakespeare summed up the final stage well in his *Seven Ages of Man*: we go back to a kind of second childhood, where we are not fully capable mentally. This may be quite mild, where the patient is known to be a little "dotty" (short for dotage), or as severe as full-blown dementia. The "Seventh Age" applies to women also. Women tend to suffer more from the dementias.

> **There are approximately 100 billion brain cells (neurones), each making between 5,000 and 50,000 hard-wired connections or "synapses".**

You do not want to enter this final stage, for sure. Many people dread losing their faculties as they get older and even, half jokingly, ask someone to put a bullet to their head, rather than allow this to happen, so great is the abhorrence of becoming mentally inept.

I urge you to follow the advice given throughout this book and with luck, you never will. Age-related deterioration of the brain is not inevitable, as many lucid centegenarians prove, so don't buy into this mind set. Treasure yourself and be determined to go on and on, enjoying life to the full, right to the very end.

Facts You May Not Know

The human brain has been described as the "3 pound universe", meaning that all our thoughts, actions, perceptions, emotions, desires, and dreams are contained in an organ weighing no more than 50 ounces, lodged inside the skull! There are approximately 100 billion brain cells (neurones), each making between 5,000 and 50,000 hard-wired connections or "synapses".

That means around 4 quadrillion connections! This awesome power needs a great deal of energy (a total of 25 watts, for those who are technically minded). In fact, our brain, which is only 2% of body weight, requires 25-30% of our nutritional energy output. That makes the brain very vulnerable to damage and degeneration, from lack of oxygen, poor nutrition, toxic overload and chemical deposits, including drugs. It means we have to look after our brain with extra care.

The good news is that a the age of 75, you still have 85% of the brain cells that you were born with, and scientists at the Salk Institute in La Jolla, California have now proven that brain cells can replace themselves. Previously it was always thought that loss of brain cells was permanent, but we can now potentially regenerate and revitalize our brains. This is great to know.

Therefore, the more we can look after our diet, take the right nutrients and keep our minds active – the better our brain's will work.

What You Can Do

The first point to grasp is that your brain thrives on activity! It's a use it or lose it thing. Science has shown that the number of connections in the brain can be increased, no matter the starting point, by simply making demands of the mind. More connections mean more brainpower. Any kind of stimulus is valid, be it crosswords, conversation, creative hobbies, sports or the arts, but doing what you love has the most benefits.

Daily exercise is also important. It stimulates and tones up both body and mind. You know the old saying "healthy body equals healthy mind". I couldn't agree more. Exercise releases endorphins, increases circulation, and therefore oxygen supply to the brain. Endorphins are natural feel-good substances in our bodies.

Don't just think in terms of swimming, jogging or cycling. Walking is very good and non-stressful. Dancing is even better, since it has the added joy element, which reminds us we are young at heart, and that life after all is great!

See also Chapter 14.

Balancing your hormones can also help return brain function to more youthful levels. See under Hormones and the related sections.

Alzheimer's Disease

Trust me. You don't want Alzheimer's. Don't suppose you'll be "gone" and not know what's happening to you. People with a good degree of recovery (yes, it happens and I'll share with you how) have returned to tell us it is unpleasant.

There are presently an estimated 5 million Alzheimer's patients in the US alone; other developed countries, like the UK, follow proportionately. Experts are estimating that within 30 years more than half of the population over 85 will suffer with Alzheimer's disease.

Drug treatment is controversial (which means basically useless); tacrine (Cognex) the most widely prescribed drug has been refused licensing in several countries, since there is no evidence it does any good, despite aggressive marketing persuading doctors to prescribe it. Sadly, a number of drugs are known to make the problem worse, such as L-Dopa and acetaminophen (Tylenol).

Beware phony societies like the Alzheimer's Association. They pretend to be offering "advice" about Alzheimer's when in fact they are simply pushing the drugs and blocking natural therapies. I was once scheduled to speak to the Alzheimer's Association and it was stopped, because I was going to talk about nutrition!

Their website states that: "At this time, there is no treatment to cure, delay, or stop the progression of Alzheimer's disease. FDA-approved drugs temporarily slow worsening of symptoms for about 6 to 12 months, on average, for about half of the individuals who take them." Yet still they promote the drug approach and refuse to admit there is any evidence of effective management using natural resources.

The truth is that Alzheimer's is a preventable disease and can even be reversed to a degree, sometimes remarkably so. One has to approach it the right way.

Risk Factors

Certain studies have shown that exposure to electromagnetic radiation significantly increases the risk of Alzheimer, or makes it rapidly worse. This means working with or near computers, VDUs and similar equipment. Also, it means that mobile phones are adding to the risk.

> **Drug treatment is controversial (which means basically useless).**

Good scientific studies have tied Alzheimer's disease to plasma homocysteine levels. Increased amounts of this important biomarker in the blood spells trouble for the heart and brain. However, homocysteine levels can be readily brought to normal, using vitamin B6, B12 and folic acid supplements. I usually add TMG (trimethyl glycine) 1,000 mgms daily. Very few doctors' approach important diseases from a nutritional perspective, yet in this case it can be wonderfully helpful.

An important study at Heidelberg University showed that a large proportion of Alzheimer's cases are the result of failure of small blood vessels in the brain (this would lead to brain starvation and degeneration). An important modern treatment, chelation, is known to be very good at restoring the function of older blood vessels.

Dementia does sometimes improve, after chelation, sometimes remarkably well.

Another part of the puzzle could be exposure to toxic metal poisoning. Aluminum was thought to be a main offender. Actually, fewer people think that today. Mercury poisoning seems a far more likely culprit, according to studies carried out at a Texas hospital.

But whichever is correct, the good news is that chelation can remove these toxic metals from the tissues. This has been done effectively for over fifty years. Modern switched-on doctors have recognized the value of chelation for Alzheimer's and other degenerative disorders caused by metal poisoning.

Diet Changes

You're probably tired of reading each section banging on about diet. But what you eat is critical to everything, especially how energetic you feel.

Food allergy and intolerance affects how you think. We talk of brain allergies and my amazing discoveries of these effects were one of the main ways I rose to fame in the 1980s.

In his *Anatomy of Melancholy* (1621) Robert Burton, an English cleric noted: "Milk, and all that comes of milk, as butter and cheese, curds etc., increase melancholy." It is the first recorded recognition that food intolerance could cause depression. Since then it has become abundantly clear that many foods can and do have this selective adverse effect in intolerant individuals.

But depression isn't the only symptom.

A doctor friend of mine, who regarded himself to be in perfect health, did some experimental testing on himself to discover whether he had any food allergies. He uncovered an allergy to wheat. As a further test, he omitted wheat from his diet.

To his surprise, he no longer felt tired at the end of a busy day and woke in the morning with a feeling of exhilaration instead of his usual dread of a heavy day's work. The doctor suddenly realised that his perfect health was far from being as good as it could be.

When bread, which is usually regarded as the staff of life, disagrees with you, and you are an unsuspecting victim of what is happening, as a consequence you can come to regard health as a mere absence of disease.

A positive sense of well-being with plenty of energy always ready for use is what should be regarded as normal health.

An allergy to the food you are eating everyday can take the edge off your enjoyment of life, and it can cause you to feel years older than you need to, without anything definite to complain about or can actually be the cause of severe inexplicable illness.

Food allergy has been well described as the unsuspected enemy. Because this source of illness tends to remain unsuspected, it is a pleasant surprise to discover how easy it can be to get well, once the possibility of food allergy is taken into consideration.

It is usual to think of food allergy in terms of the type of illness, which results from an allergy to strawberries or to shellfish. These foods however are not eaten on a day-to-day basis, and the violence of the reaction leaves little opportunity for the source of the illness to remain unsuspected. There is a marked reaction to the food, which dies down and disappears within a short time.

But there is an entirely different clinical picture when the food to which you are allergic is a staple item of your diet that you eat every day of your life, perhaps several times each day.

Under these circumstances, the body adapts to the allergic process and the reaction disappears to become a masked allergy. This adaptation of the body may last a lifetime or may become exhausted at any time under stress. When the adaption by the body is complete, there are no symptoms, but if the strain of coping with the allergy wears down the adaptive process then a whole variety of symptoms may break surface.

At different times in a person's life, these breakthrough manifestations of the underlying masked allergy may present themselves in a wide variety of illnesses.

Indeed, one of the main characteristics of illness due to food allergy is the wide variety of symptoms. Any bodily system can be upset by food allergy and in any one patient one or more systems can be involved. The system involved can change from one period of life to another.

An allergy to food and chemicals seems to guarantee an adverse reaction to drugs and medicines, the patient tends to get worse and becomes a very difficult case ending up allergic to almost everything.

In a typical case of masked food allergy, the patient may suffer mainly from involvement of the central nervous system. Perhaps the most distressing symptom of all is what has been described by patients as the woolly brain syndrome ("brain fog").

An inability to concentrate, a confusion of thinking, an impairment of memory and a tendency to just sit in an inactive torpor, are all symptoms, which cause great distress to a patient who is normally highly intelligent, very industrious and exceptionally competent. Depression is a common and distressing symptom. I have often heard patients with this complaint say that they would kill themselves if they could only bring themselves to do it. Life becomes intolerable.

This state of affairs can put an impossible strain on a marriage. In this condition, the person does not wish to be touched and may turn nasty in response to any sort of advance from the marital partner.

These patients often come to be labelled neurotic hypochondriacs and because they cannot explain or understand their own predicament they often come to believe themselves to be insane or going insane. Once these patients are put on drugs, and become addicted to drugs the true state of affairs is virtually impossible to untangle and many must be ending their days in mental hospitals.

It is essential that patients suffering from lack of energy, cognitive impairment, general slowing down, and symptoms of mental dysfunction be investigated competently for the possibility of toxic and allergic food reactions. The bench mark is elimination and challenge eating but there are many pitfalls in this seemingly simple procedure, which will confuse the unwary. Once again, I refer you to my book "Diet Wise".

Treatment For Alzheimer's
It is vital to understand that all good general health issues are also good news for a tired and deteriorating brain. Exercise, sound nutrition, and avoidance of stress are all critical factors.

But certain specific treatments have been shown to be highly beneficial. For example, one study showed that vitamin E was better than drug or placebo in reducing the symptoms of Alzheimer's. The values of B6, B12, and folate have already been alluded to above.

There are two powerful substances, which generate nerve growth factor. That leads to an increase in the number of available neurons and neurites in the brain.

The substance I recommend unreservedly is the lion's mane mushroom, *Hericium erinaceous*. There is a lot science backing up the fact that this mushroom is capable of enhancing brain structure and activity, via nerve growth factors. Clinically, I know of one severe case where the patient cured himself completely by eating lots of this mushroom (it grows freely in the forest).

Gotu Kola has also been shown to increase neurogenesis (see below).

In a very important study published in 1997 by the Journal of the American Medical Association, Gingko Biloba was shown not only to prevent Alzheimer's degeneration but actually improved many of the cases, compared to the placebo (all the more remarkable, in that the AMA has always been opposed to natural and nutritional therapies!)

Also helpful are glutathione, N-acetyl cysteine, and alpha lipoic acid. These are powerful brain anti-oxidants and have remarkable effects on mental performance and cognition. So much so that otherwise healthy individuals notice considerable improvement too!

IV Anti-Oxidant Therapy

This is a name I invented for my variation of IV chelation.

It is a specially compounded formula, based on chelation, administered intravenously (as a drip) weekly on an outpatient basis (takes around 2 hours). It is quite painless and easy. There are now literally hundreds of thousands of successful chelation cases, attesting to its safety and effectiveness. Its ability to remove toxic damaging metals has been pointed out. It also can reverse age-deterioration. Specifically, it can reverse the cross-linkage of proteins that leads to wrinkles, stiffness, and poor movement function.

Following the groundbreaking work of Dr. David Perlmutter in the USA, it is appropriate to add glutathione, which is administered intravenously. He has observed what he calls the "glutathione miracle" and seen patients with severe Parkinson's disease within one hour be able to stand, walk, and move their arms around normally. Perlmutter has used glutathione extensively in cases with Alzheimer's and other dementias, multiple sclerosis, strokes and ME. Interestingly, glutathione administered this way stops diarrhea and irritable bowel disease in its tracks.

When I introduced it to my regime, I noticed the same startling effects. One patient recovered the use of an arm and hand, *even though he had been paralyzed by a stroke 30 years earlier!*

Good website to visit: BrainRecovery.com. Dr David Perlmutter's book of the same title is also highly recommended (ISBN 0-9635874-1-2)

Incidentally, Dr. Perlmutter now uses pioglitazone ("Pio") against brain inflammatory degeneration. In his blog, I see he has quoted studies showing that Pio-treated transgenic mice revealed improved muscle strength and body weight, exhibited a delayed disease onset, and survived significantly longer than non-treated mice.

Quantification of motor neurons of the spinal cord at day 90 revealed complete neuroprotection by Pio, whereas non-treated mice had lost 30% of motor neurons. Also, activated microglia (so-called glial plaques) were significantly reduced at sites of neurodegeneration in Pio-treated mice.

Sounds a good possibility but you'll need to get an MD to work on this for you.

Brain Saver Supplements
Alpha-Lipoic Acid and Acetyl-L-Carnitine

Glutathione is manufactured in our cells from a number of precursors such as Alpha Lipoic Acid (**ALA**); Acetyl- L – Carnitine and N-Acetyl Cysteine (NAC).

In a 2002 published study, rats fed on extra ALA and Acetyl-L-Carnitine lived 50% longer than normal rats and enjoyed greatly improved overall health. The animals were so vigorous that media headlines referred to the "dancing rats". The evidence is so convincing that the scientists concerned have patented the mixture but there is nothing to stop you benefitting personally from this breakthrough.

Acetyl L-Carnitine (ALC) is a nutrient that also stimulates the brain to produce nerve growth factors. ALC increases the effects of nerve growth factor, which acts to re-grow neurites and dendrites. Neurites are the nerve fibers that enable brain cells to connect with each and function effectively. Loss of this network during your life can lead to memory loss and degenerative diseases like Parkinson's and Alzheimer's.

> [Barhwal K, Hota SK, Jain V, Prasad D, Singh SB, Ilavazhagan G (June 2009). "Acetyl-l-carnitine (ALCAR) prevents hypobaric hypoxia-induced spatial memory impairment through extracellular related kinase-mediated nuclear factor erythroid 2-related factor 2 phosphorylation." Neuroscience 161 (2): 501-14].

The best sources of ALC are grass-fed beef, poultry, fish, and dairy products. Fruits, vegetables, and grains contain relatively little.

You can also get ALA and ALC in supplement form at your local vitamin shop or health food store. I recommend taking 500 mg twice a day on an empty stomach.

After the age of 50 we suggest you take 200mg of ALA, and 500mg of either NAC or Acetyl L Carnitine on a daily basis. For someone with Alzheimer's you can try doubling the ALC to 500 mgm twice a day (taken on an empty stomach).

Phosphatidyl Choline and Serine

Phosphatidyl serine and phosphatidyl choline help to protect nerve fibers and keep the brain fit and sleek -   take a minimum of 50mg daily or either, or both. Lecithin—derived from soya beans—is rich in phosphatidyl serine and choline. A teaspoon of the granules daily (make sure they contain at least 30% PS or PC) not only helps increase memory but also reduces LDL, the 'bad' cholesterol.

Gotu Kola

Gotu Kola is a slender, creeping plant that grows commonly in swampy areas of Sri Lanka, where you may know I lived for some years. It also grows in nearby India, Madagascar, South Africa, and the tropics. Its fan shaped leaves are about the size of an old British penny - hence its common names Indian pennywort, marsh penny, and water pennywort.

Putting back the growth factors that decline with age is the best way to slow down the shrinking of the brain and Gotu Kola can do that, we now know, thanks to a new study. Gotu Kola extract helped increase neurite growth in human brain cells. [Garcia-Alloza M, Dodwell SA, Meyer-Leuhmann, M Hyman BT, Bacskai BJ. "Plaque-derived oxidative stress mediates distorted neurite trajectories in the Alzheimer mouse model." J Neuropathol Exp Neuro. 2006 Nov;65(11): 1082-9]

Here are three of the most common ways to take Gotu Kola:

1. As an extract, like the one used in the study. Take 10 drops per day.
2. As a dried herb. You can make a tea of the dried leaf, three times daily.
3. As a powdered herb (available in capsules). Take 400-600 mg, three times a day.

Ginkgo Biloba

This herb needs no introduction; it's so well known.

There is good science to show it can improve memory, increase circulation, and acts as a brain stimulant.

Dose: 500mg of standardized extract daily. Remember that herbs are potent medicines and not always without side effects - take for 6 weeks, then stop for a month and then begin again.

Ginseng

This plant extract contains many good things to feed the brain. Special glycosides improve cerebral blood flow and work as stimulants of certain neurotransmitters, chemical messengers the brain uses to send out signals.

Ginseng helps regulate blood sugar and so is of benefit in reducing the insulin resistance-diabetes progression. It also has benefits for the thymus gland and spleen, thus making it a great all-round anti-ager. Ginseng is taken as teas, powders, and capsules; the quality varies greatly.

> **Ginseng helps regulate blood sugar and so is of benefit in reducing the insulin resistance-diabetes progression.**

Avoid its strong tone-up action if you already have blood pressure or heart disease (go for kava instead, which is a relaxant).

Vinpocetine
I left one of the best till last!

This substance is an extract of the wonder plant Vinca minor (periwinkle); from the same source we also get two anti-cancer chemo-therapeutic agents

(vinblastine and vincristine).

In humans vinpocetine has been shown to:

- dilate brain arteries (more nutrients)
- reduce the tendency of blood to clot (thus protecting against heart disease and stroke)
- speed up brain metabolism
- act as an antioxidant
- aid recovery after stroke

In a 1985 Japanese study, vinpocetine helped two thirds of stroke patients recover rapidly, *even when administered years after the original stroke.* A 1987 study in the *Journal of the American Geriatric Society* showed unequivocally that vinpocetine protects against dementia and improves those who already have it. Good enough reasons for vinpocetine to be classed as a major anti-aging substance.

Other Brain Nutrients
I paraphrase what I said about anti-aging in general: *All good health measures are good brain preserving methods.*

Any health and recovery plan will work better when there is general sound nutrition. Never forget to add a multi vitamin/mineral formula that contains at least 500mg of vitamin C, 25mg of B6, and 25mg of B1 and 100mcg of B12.

Also 300mg of magnesium, which is known as "Nature's Tranquillizer". A deficiency of magnesium has a detrimental effect on a huge array of enzyme reactions, which take place in our bodies, many of them related to the energy-building cycle of metabolism that takes place in the mitochondria.

The brain is one of the first organs to feel the lack. Magnesium also helps prevent diabetes, blood pressure, irregular heart, headaches, osteoporosis, and many other conditions you would recognize simply as a catalogue of aging!

Folic Acid Helps Prevent Cognitive Decline
A new study, published in the Lancet Jan 20th 2007, has shown daily folic acid significantly improves cognitive performance in older adults — specifically as it relates to memory and information processing.

A randomized, placebo-controlled trial, which included 818 subjects aged 50 to 70 years who were folate deficient, showed that those who took 800 μg daily of oral folic acid for 3 years had significantly better memory and information processing speed than subjects in the placebo group. Furthermore, serum folate concentrations increased by 576% and plasma total homocysteine concentrations decreased by 26% in participants taking folic acid compared with those taking placebo (homocysteine is an inflammation marker and you want its levels down).

"Word fluency was not affected by folic acid supplementation, perhaps because encyclopedic memory is a component of crystallized intelligence that stays relatively intact as one grows older," the authors write. [Lancet. 2007;369:208-216].

Hormones and Brain Function

Here follows one of the most important and yet least attended aspects of maintaining brain function: hormones. As you know, these vital life substances affect all aspects of the running and performance of our bodies and that applies equally to the brain.

Unfortunately, doctors dealing with aging, depression, dementia and other aspects of neurological decline often ignore the great impact of these substances on our mental well-being.

Yet omitting to test hormones in a mentally dysfunctional patient is as negligent as not taking an x-ray of a patient who has been badly injured in a fall. Once hormone deficiencies have been proven, then they can be easily corrected, often resulting in enormous benefit. The aim is to have a hormone profile similar to that of a healthy young person. Sometimes this alone lifts the depression completely and with lasting effect.

See Chapter 10 for more understanding on hormones.

More Supplements With Specific Mood-Boosting Benefits

Phenylethylamine (PEA). This compound is an endogenous neuroamine and has been called the "love molecule". PEA unquestionably increases mood and leads to sustained relief of depression in a significant number of patients. PEA works as rapidly as amphetamine but does not produce tolerance. [Sabelli H, Fink P, Fawcett J, et al. Sustained antidepressant effects of PEA replacement. J Neuropsychiatry 1996;8:168–.71]. It is found in chocolate but highest concentrations are found in the blue-green algae *Aphanizomenon flos-aquae* (AFA).

Recommended dose: aim for about 800 mgms of AFA.

PEA is also present in good healthy chocolate and one of the reported "side effects" of my "Doctor's Chocolate, is that people feel much more cheerful and some patients have been able to throw away their anti-depressants! Eat more good chocolate (you can order mine here):

www.thedoctorschocolate.com

Phenylalanine

This is related to PEA and a number of studies have shown it to be similarly effective in raising mood. It leads to an increase in the body's natural PEA levels (measured by urinary excretion). Side effects are few and include mild headache, low blood pressure, and agitation.

Phenylalanine may also help regulate disordered glucose metabolism, which we have already seen is implicated in the aging process. [Journal of Orthomolecular Psychiatry (Regina) 5(3):199-202, 1976 and Biological Psychiatry 10(2):235-239, 1975]

Take 200-500 mg daily of phenylalanine.

S-Adenosyl methionine (SAMe)

Another great mood-booster.

SAMe (pronounced sammy) has long been known as an effective antidepressant in its own right and is widely prescribed by doctors in Europe. Clinical trials comparing both oral and intramuscular forms of SAMe to tricyclic antidepressants show SAMe to be as effective as tricyclic antidepressants in reducing the symptoms of depression (Mischoulon D et al 2002; Pancheri P et al 2002). SAMe is associated with fewer adverse events (Pancheri P et al 2002) and is better tolerated than conventional antidepressants (Delle CR et al 2002).

See LE Magazine June 2003: A New Era for SAMe for more details of this amazing health-giving nutrient.

Take 100-400 mg of SAMe daily without food. If you are feeling depressed, this can rise to 400-1,200 mg.

Tryptophan and 5-hydroxytryptophan (5HT)

Available as dietary supplements, these two substances are immediate precursors to serotonin. Serotonin, we all know, is what makes us feel happy! We need plenty. These precursors are good for enhancing serotonin levels (Murphy SE et al 2006). This may be a better plan than taking St. John's Wort as a serotonin preserver.

Tryptophan is very safe, whatever the FDA claims. You may know that in 1989, the use of dietary supplements containing tryptophan was blamed for the development of a serious condition called eosinophilia-myalgia syndrome (EMS), which caused severe muscle and joint pain, high fever, weakness, swelling of the arms and legs, and shortness of breath in more than a thousand people. In addition, more than 30 deaths were attributed to EMS caused by tryptophan supplements.

It seems clear that the EMS was caused by a contaminant that was found in one batch of tryptophan sold by one manufacturer and occurred in only a small number of susceptible individuals. However, the United States Food and Drug Administration, remained convinced that high doses of tryptophan were categorically unsafe. Since 1989, tryptophan has not been available as a dietary supplement in the United States.

Try 500 to 1000 mg of tryptophan once or twice daily on an empty stomach.

Dr. Keith special insights

Eat Chocolate

Chocolate is good for the brain. It increases blood flow and that's great.

Ian Macdonald of Britain's University of Nottingham Medical School, conducted a small brain imaging study on young, healthy women to see whether flavonols -rich cocoa helped boost cognitive function during challenging mental tasks.

Although it did not measurably improve their performance on the tests, it did increase blood flow to their brains for a two to three-hour period, Macdonald said. I'm not sure how much cognitive function increase he expected to see in just a few hours.

But the researchers believed more research might show that increased blood flow could benefit older adults and those who have cognitive impairments, such as fatigue or even mini-strokes. That's quite logical.

A U.S. study of healthy adults over 50 also found a marked rise in blood flow to the brain. Harvard Medical School researcher, Dr. Norman Hollenberg, who studied the effects of cocoa and flavonols on Panama's Kuna Indian population, conducted it. This increase in blood flow to the brain fits with what I was telling you about relaxing blood vessels and improving blood viscosity.

My own "Doctor's Chocolate" is naturally a boast. Listen to a 40-minute audio here, describing its (many) health and longevity virtues. You can find a link there to purchase and try some. Delicious!

Carnitine

Is a supplement that has been shown repeatedly to increase energy levels, boost low moods, and promote weight loss through its effect on fat and glucose metabolism. Men take special note that carnitine may be equal to testosterone in its ability to improve sexual function. [Cavallini G, Caracciolo S, Vitali G, Modenini F, Biagiotti G. Carnitine versus androgen administration in the treatment of sexual dysfunction, depressed mood, and fatigue associated with male aging. Urology. 2004 Apr;63(4):641-6].

Carnitine is safe and effective at levels of 2,000-3,000 mgm daily.

Surprise! More out of the box...

Vitamin D Cognitive Function

Vitamin D does so much; it goes way beyond preventing rickets. We know it plays a role in cancer prevention, priming immune function, bettering heart disease and has even been suggested as a buffer against autism (when loaded with vitamin D, some children have made remarkable recoveries).

Now there may be a similar role in adult cognitive function.

Katherine Tucker, from Tufts University (Massachusetts, USA), and colleagues studied more than 1,000 men and women, ages 65 to 99 years, receiving home care, assessing vitamin D blood levels (measured as 25-hydroxyvitamin D, or 25(OH)D) and conducting neuropsychological tests.

Those with adequate vitamin D scored significantly higher on tests of cognitive performance, particularly on measures of "executive performance," such as cognitive flexibility, perceptual complexity, and reasoning, as compared to those in the deficient and insufficient categories.

What was perhaps shocking was that only 35% of the patients had adequate healthy vitamin D blood levels.

[Jennifer S. Buell, Tammy M. Scott, Bess Dawson-Hughes, Gerard E. Dallal, Irwin H. Rosenberg, Marshal F. Folstein, Katherine L. Tucker. "Vitamin D Is Associated With Cognitive Function in Elders Receiving Home Health Services." J Gerontol A Biol Sci Med Sci, 2009 64A(8): 888-895; doi:10.1093/gerona/glp032.]

Be sure to supplement vitamin D (as D3) at a minimum of 2,000 IU daily. Up to 4,000 is quite safe and even then may barely bring a deficient person up to correct nutritional status of this remarkable and versatile vitamin.

12 | Look After Your Skin

Nothing gives away our age quite so much as wrinkles, especially of the face - fine lines at the outer corner of the smile lines of the eyes (known as crow's feet). Thinning and loss of tone to the skin is one of the hallmarks of the aging process.

Can we do anything about it? You bet.

First, any good anti-aging measure is good for the skin and complexion. Number one among those I would put a healthy diet. It needs to be constructed on a person-by-person basis, working out the foods, which suit you personally. I explain the importance of this in Chapter 5.

Diet

There is no question in my mind that the number one cosmetic for women (and men) is a good healthy diet.

All natural foods, organic if you can get it, with lashings of anti-oxidants is about as good as it gets. That will hold back your wrinkles a lot longer than growth hormone, DHEA or anything else in the remainder of this book.

Once again, I have to add the caveat from Chapter 5: any food can be a stress food. Whatever I recommend here is subject to the fact that you can tolerate it well.

But in general foods of the Mediterranean Diet type are good for the skin. The wrinkly old Greek grannies and browned farmers of Provence that you see so commonly have wrinkled skin because of the intense sunshine, not because the food doesn't work for skin.

The Mediterranean Diet isn't just a diet; it's a lifestyle. After all, it was the nutrition of an entire culture. It's the best way to prevent all kinds of diseases such as myocardial infarction (heart attack), stroke, or brain ictus. While we won't go into detail about the diet, itself the general characteristics are:

1. High consumption of virgin olive oil.
2. High intake of vegetables, fruits, and legumes.
3. One or two small glasses of red wine a day.
4. Use of non refined carbohydrates.
5. Consumption of milk and derivates, cheese and yogurt but not too much.

6. Three eggs per week.
7. Consumption of fish, specially oily at least three times a week.
8. Moderate consumption of meat and saturated fats.
9. Nuts as snacks.

Wine Is Good!

Resveratrol, we know, is good for the heart. But it's great for the skin too. Before you rush out for nips and tucks or the dreaded Botox, consider a glass of something mellow and fruitful: red wine!

According to plastic surgeon Richard A. Baxter, MD, a plastic surgeon in Seattle and the author of Age Gets Better with Wine, a glass or two of wine a day is good for beauty!

There is quite a lot of data on the wine and beauty connection. Again, they key to this is the antioxidant content of red wine. There is a much higher concentration of healthful antioxidants called polyphenols in wine compared to grape juice. In wine, the skin and seeds are part of the fermenting process, but both are removed when making grape juice.

I think stress busting also has something to do with it, too. It is difficult to sort out how much of the benefits are from the chemical properties of wine vs. the types of behaviors that wine drinkers tend to have. Wine relaxes and creates camaraderie. That is good at reducing stress. Less stress means less aging. It's all circular!

> **Drinking a glass of red wine a day could be the single most important thing that you can do other than nonsmoking.**

Wine is part of the Mediterranean diet, which is also rich in fresh fruits and vegetables, whole grains, nuts and seeds, legumes, seafood, yogurt, and olive oil. This diet is more of a lifestyle that includes drinking wine with dinner. Studies show that the Mediterranean diet is associated with longer, healthier lives.

Drinking a glass of red wine a day could be the single most important thing that you can do other than nonsmoking, from an anti-aging point of view! You can have too much of a good thing, of course. Drinking more than recommended can have the opposite effect on your appearance and health.

How much? A glass a day and your skin will glow, says Dr. Baxter. You will look better, your skin will glow, and you will live five years longer than a teetotaler. There are also good studies that show people who drink red wine on a regular basis have fewer actinic keratoses [precancerous skin lesions].

You will have a significantly lower risk of Alzheimer's disease, cancer, diabetes, and all of the things that go along with aging. People assume that drinking would decrease brainpower as you get old, but the most amazing thing is that regular wine drinkers have an 80% lower risk of developing Alzheimer's disease.

As anti-aging advice, this is as good as it gets.

If You Can't Drink Alcohol, Eat Chocolate!

What about people who can't consume alcohol?

People who can't or don't drink wine should such look to other whole foods with polyphenols and antioxidants, like pomegranates and blueberries. Or go for dark chocolate. It does a lot of the same things as wine. Both dark chocolate and red wine have been shown to protect the skin from sun damage.

The ladies, I know, would love to hear that chocolate is good for the skin. It helps protect against skin cancer and will prevent the signs of aging in the skin. The Journal of Nutrition June 2006 reported a German study, which involved 24 women who added hot cocoa to their breakfasts daily for about three months.

Half-received cocoa that contained 329 milligrams of flavonols while the rest received a placebo cocoa that contained only 27 mg of flavonols per serving. Those with all the flavonols had 25% less skin reddening after UV light exposure after 3 months.

These ladies also had a doubling of blood flow in the skin in tissue and a 37.5% increase in tissue. Since the main aging effect in skin, which leads to wrinkles, is that it goes thinner with age and loses collagen, this is great news and totally the opposite of what you thought!

For the best health chocolate in the world, I am naturally inclined to recommend my own designer chocolate""The Doctor's Chocolate". You can watch some videos, learn more and get some to try here:

http://www.doctorkeithschocolate.com

Botox

We all know what this is. It's a toxin (Botulinum toxin). It works by paralyzing the nerves to the face; those which cause expression and wrinkles.

There are several problems with this treatment:

- It can go wrong and produce deformity, even in skilled hands.
- After a while it stops working. By this stage most of the facial muscles are paralyzed anyway. It is very limited.
- You will have a mask like face. You'll wish you hadn't done it by this time but it's irreversible.

People still do it but this pathway to block aging is silly and does nothing to increase your health or extend life. It's just papering over the cracks, not rejuvenating or restorative.

Homeopathic Botox (Better!)

This is not a homeopathic preparation of Botulinum toxin but a completely different formula. A preparation called MADE was developed by **Ma**ssimo **De**belli of Italy (hence it's name) and it is quite logical. It contains all kinds of good tissue energizing and nourishing substances, all harmless.

MADE is intended to be injected, at select acupuncture sites around the face, rather like mesotherapy.

I learned it a few years ago from Debelli himself, in Milan, Italy.

It is normally done bi-weekly and can be continued and/or repeated as often as you like.

Homeopathic Botox does not produce the rapid and disastrous destruction of normal facial tissue. Rather, it gently encourages regeneration and restoration of skin tissues.

You can have it as often as you like and for as long as you feel it works for you. Botox, of course, has a strict limit. When every muscle in your face is paralyzed, there is no point in going further!

Chelation

One of the more dramatic effects of EDTA chelation therapy is the diminishment of wrinkles and a return of softer, more supple looking skin. I can confirm this from my own work at my London Anti-Aging clinic.

The late Dr. Charlie Farr, from Oklahoma, performed studies that supports this happy finding. Before he began treating a group of older patients with chelation therapy, he took samples of skin from their arms. He discovered that the common stiffness and dryness they experienced with age was a result of cross-linkages of calcium. Following chelation therapy he noticed the cross linkages were gone, and his patients were reporting softer, smoother skin.

Aging involves hard arteries and soft bones. The process of aging is what researchers and doctors call calcinosis, meaning calcium is pulled from the bones and deposited into soft tissue, settling in your arteries, joints and skin, causing arthritis and the pale, hard, wrinkled look of aging.

Calcium deposits can also cause strokes and circulation problems. What chelation therapy does is remove calcium from the soft tissues, where it doesn't belong, and puts it hack into the bones, where it does belong.

In other words, chelation can increase bone density.

For maximum benefit, EDTA therapy should be accompanied by a carefully tailored program of vitamin and mineral supplements. This is because of the delicate balance of nutrients and the body's use of calcium. For example, those with low intakes of vitamin D have higher parathyroid function in the winter. The parathyroid glands draw on calcium reserves in the bone to keep blood levels normal. Parahormone is the hormone excreted by the parathyroid glands, which control calcium and phosphorus metabolism.

For more on the fascinating, enlightening and underrated preventive and healing effects of chelation therapy, especially against aging, read the book, Forty Something Forever by Harold and Arlene Brecher. We're only as old as our arteries. Drink from this Fountain of Youth and be young again!

Find a certified chelation doctor at the American College For The Advancement Of Medicine (ACAM: http://www.acam.org).

Hyaluronic Acid (Ha)

HA is a special mucopolysaccharide that is the normal lubricant in human joints. When present in a joint, even one with minimal or no cartilage, it provides a cushion effect. It is also part of connective tissue and joins cells together.

Aging causes the hyaluronic acid in the skin to decrease, leaving the skin dry and wrinkled. Replenishing the HA levels in the body allow the skin to retain moisture, leaving the skin soft, supple, and wrinkle-free. It is used in many cosmetics such as make-up and moisturizing creams.

Synthovial 7™ by Longevity Plus is Hyaluronic Acid (HA). The dose is one drop a day (3 mgm) in a glass of water. www.longevityplus.com

Skin Creams And Unguents

Skin creams try to prevent wrinkling and aging have a long and honorable tradition. Unfortunately, most of them are a marketing success, rather than scientifically backed.

Instant wrinkle removers contain a variety of different ingredients. Some of them succeed because of special pigments that reduce the "shadows" caused by those folds of skin. So, they are not actually healing wrinkles. It's more like they are "hiding" them.

Only phony products include collagen. Collagen molecules are too large to be absorbed by your skin, so applying collagen to your skin is a waste of time and money.

If the skin cream doesn't contain a special pigment, it will probably include some kind of acid. GABA is a popular ingredient for these products.

GABA is a neurotransmitter produced by humans and other mammals. It is responsible for regulating muscle tone. The "idea" behind including it in instant wrinkle removers is that it will relax the tiny facial muscles, although it has never been tested for effectiveness.

Neither has it been tested for safety in cosmetics by an industry panel. That's according to the Environmental Working Group's database for cosmetic ingredients.

As a word of caution, you should avoid any products that contain oxybenzone or benzophenone. These organic sun-screening compounds are supposed to protect skin from the free radical damage caused by sunlight. But independent tests shown them both to *increase free radical production and activity*. Thus, they are probable carcinogens and any ingredient that can cause cancer is counterproductive in a skincare product.

Confused? Don't know where to start?

Well, I do know a range of fabulous skin creams that prevent wrinkling. My wife Vivien swears by them and that's good enough for most of my readers, it seems (if you've ever seen pictures of how young and lovely she looks, you'll know why her recommendation carries authority!)

Enter Al Sears MD

Dr Al Sears has spent years bringing out skin care products, based on the very latest science. For example, his "Silk" is based around resveratrol. As American viewers saw on an edition of the program "60 Minutes", research has shown clearly resveratrol is good for skin as well as the heart.

If you take it only as a supplement, you're missing out on what it offers your skin, but rub resveratrol directly on your face, and it quickly goes to work. The problem is resveratrol has limited stability and water solubility. So, converting it to a "usable" topical form that can actually help over-stressed skin can be a bit tricky.

You see, the problem is most products don't penetrate deep enough to make a difference.

To maintain young-looking skin, the nutrients you rub on your face need to reach something called the "DEJ," or dermal-epidermal junction, a ridged area connecting the inner layer of skin (dermis) and your outer layer of skin (epidermis).

As your skin ages, the DEJ starts to flatten out. When that happens, the outer layer can't get enough blood flow to the inner layer, which means your skin isn't able to properly repair itself and so it becomes fragile and more prone to wrinkles.

Regular anti-aging creams don't effectively help with the appearance of wrinkles and other visible signs of aging, because their ingredients aren't potent or stable enough to reach the DEJ.

But this new and usable form of topical resveratrol, called "metrabiotics resveratrol" changes that. It's the breakthrough behind Al's new rejuvenating cream **SILK**.

Studies show the metrabiotics resveratrol found in SILK:

- Improved the look of wrinkles: **Up by 61%**
- Improvement in definition of lips: **Up by 70%**
- Better skin complexion: **Up by 61%**
- Improved the look of lines around the lips: **Up by 55%**
- Improved wrinkles and fine lines around the eyes: **Up by 51%**

There's no doubt… the people using this new kind of topical resveratrol looked and felt younger. You will see a reduction in the appearance of wrinkles and dark spots and the fine lines around your eyes… *all in less than a month when you use SILK.*

Order SILK here, right NOW and see this for yourself:

http://www.on2url.com/app/adtrack.asp?MerchantID=132773&AdID=496515

What Not To Allow On Your Skin

It's unfortunate, but women all across the globe slather dangerous chemicals on their faces every day. What you may not know is that a great deal of this stuff is absorbed directly through the skin. Of course manufacturers don't want you to know that: you'd never buy their products!

I came across research some years ago that showed women absorb up to 2 lbs of chemicals via the skin every year. That's pretty scary, when you consider what's in cosmetic products.

The ingredients in a large number of so-called "anti-aging" skincare products can damage your DNA and prevent it from repairing itself.

One of the skincare industry's biggest mistakes was PABA, an ingredient added to products to reduce the damage from the sun's UV rays. Studies performed on PABA determined in the dark it's harmless. However, expose it to sunlight, and it starts attacking your DNA. So while it may prevent you from getting sunburn, it could easily contribute to sun-related cancers.

Another ingredient found in some skin lotions and facial cleansers is ethylene glycol. According to the US Centers for Disease Control (CDC), you'll find this compound in antifreeze and de-icing solutions for cars, airplanes, and boats.

Is this really something you want to put on your face?

Here's another one you should know about: propylene glycol is an active ingredient in at least 12,080 products that touch your skin. You'll find it in cosmetics as an additive to help you retain moisture and build a moisture barrier.

Propylene glycol is often an ingredient in antifreeze, tire sealant, rubber cleaner, paint, degreasers and adhesives. Need I say more?

Telomeres Breakthrough for Skin Aging

Telomeres are the "time keepers" attached to every strand of your DNA. They're critical to youthful cell function. But each time cells divide, the telomeres get shorter eventually cell division stops and your life ends.

The telomere is the most important discovery in anti-aging. We now understand the aging mechanism and how to influence it. The discovery of telomeres won the 2009 Nobel Prize in Medicine. We can now help maintain the integrity of our DNA. We can measure telomerase, an enzyme which shows us how much telomere activity is going on.

> **The telomere is the most important discovery in human history.**

Repairing your skin's DNA, will plump up your skin and erase wrinkles, tighten up your sagging jaw line, make your crow's feet disappear, and banish sun and aging spots.

Al Sears' other major skin care product, "Revive" helps maintain telomeres and extend the lifespan of your skin cells (there are other key ingredients to help erase all of the signs of aging and revive the youth and radiance of younger years).

These potent skin-saving ingredients have real science behind them. In clinical trials of women, the results were remarkable.

Check out these numbers:

- 100% increase in the moisture in their skin
- 100% saw sun spots improve significantly
- Over 90% decrease in redness and pore size
- 75% experienced an improvement in skin tone and elasticity
- 75% felt roughness and fine lines faded noticeably

One of the significant ingredients is hyaluronic acid (HA). When you're young, you have lots but it drops off as you age. HA is one of the fillers that dermatologists inject into the skin to puff up your lips, neutralize frown lines and smooth out your skin.

There's a good reason HA is such a popular cosmetic enhancement. HA has the amazing ability to absorb around 1000 times its weight in water. Without enough moisture, your skin becomes loose, dry and wrinkled… adding years to your age.

But when your skin has enough HA, the water plumps up your skin, enhancing volume and elasticity restoring a youthful balance. You don't have to get an injection to receive the benefits of HA. Topically provides great results.

That's because your skin can absorb HA at a cellular level. HA sinks into the deeper levels of your skin tissue, unlike some others that sit on the surface.

Finally, the addition of this pure, essential oil to the "Revive" formula encourages cell regeneration and leaves your face soft and glowing for the world to see.

SCENAR Cosmetology Technique

Many of you will be aware of my enthusiasm for the Russian SCENAR device. I wrote about it in my book "Virtual Medicine" and started a SCENAR revolution in the West! Google SCENAR (sometimes spelled SKENAR) and you'll see my name come up over and over.

Just the size of a TV remote control, the SCENAR is capable of a vast range of healing potentials, including working as a defibrillator, bone setter, immune booster and anti-inflammatory. But not many readers will be aware that the SCENAR has fantastic potential in the realm of cosmetology (esthetology). It's a boon to men and women. It gets rid of wrinkles and tones up the face most remarkably.

The SCENAR can take years off your face!

Now Pacific Health Options, SCENAR suppliers in Vancouver, Canada, are offering a cosmetology package, using the home device SCENAR (you can, of course, do this with the professional model too).

Using the SCENAR or Avazzia and the instructions that come with it you will learn how to exercise each group of muscles in your face causing them to tighten removing years as the fine lines and wrinkles suddenly disappear because the skin is taught from muscles that are plumped. It's not much different than any other workout.

You can decide on what facial zones to start with by standing in front of the mirror. It's really quite simple. You'll remove all makeup otherwise you would force it deep into the skin and that's not what you want to do. When the electrodes are properly placed on your skin it will be a smooth process, however if you do not get the electrodes press on firmly there may be an uncomfortable tingling.

If you want to moisturize your skin using the SCENAR, use either a special electro conductive gel or just water.

Learn more about the cosmetology package, created just for my subscribers, here:

http://www.home-scenar.com

Star Trek Medicine

I'm credited with introducing this jokey term. Remember Dr. McCoy with his little hand-held device and his ability to grow new limbs or treat any disease? Well the SCENAR isn't quite there but you apply it to a diseased area where there is pain or injury it sends a biofeedback signal changing the pathological energies and then you will get healing.

It does a lot more than cosmetology! Dr. John Hache and Dr. Lorrain Hache were involved with SCENAR from the minute the Russians let the technology out. When it comes to SCENAR cosmetology this is impressive technology.

For example, scar tissue has a lot of pain associated with it and SCENAR when set at the right frequency allows for the destruction of scar tissue within minutes. So after seeing what it could do with scar tissue the logical question was what could it do on skin.

With SCENAR, you receive a non-invasive face lift – tightening up the muscles in the face. There will be no scar tissue formed, which is what cosmetology surgery does it creates scar tissue. Easy to use, self-treatment, after 8 to 10 treatments chest upwards, you will only have to treat the problem areas. Repetition – once you know your movements it's easy.

While you may not look 21 again you can turn back the clock to 45-50 before things start to sag and you can definitely slow down the aging process. While cosmetology devices are not regulated, the FDA authorizes this device and it is cleared as a type II medical device and a type II biofeedback device.

13 | Movement and Exercise

I have used the word movement here for a specific reason, in the way that emotion is mostly expressed as a certain action or movement. If you watch people, you will be very clear that aging too expresses mainly as movement.

Stiffness and slow movement seem to be the hallmarks of aging; we don't want that, do we? One of the great barometers of physiological age is how a person moves. Some agers are still dancing beyond the age of 100 years. Others you see around can hardly walk at the age of 60, or sometimes younger.

Take It Easy!
Remember Dr. Li Ching-Yun's formula for living to over 250 years: "Keep a quiet heart; sit like a tortoise; sleep like a dog". This accords well with modern anti-aging science, which says avoid stress, avoid inflammatory, over-exertion, and sleep at least 8 hours!

Now you will know that one of the ways to remain healthy and fit is to exercise. But I'm going way out of the box here, and I want to warn you about what I know: **excess exercising is one of the fastest ways to age there is.**

Vigorous exercise produces showers of free radicals. It also creates a flood of white cells to the peripheral blood. Conclusion: heavy exercise is highly inflammatory in character. There is faulty reasoning everywhere: because some is good, then more and more must be the way to go. That is certainly not true with exercise. You CAN have too much.

I Bet Nobody Told You That Before! But It's True.
To go out getting "ripped" as they say in modern fashion, stretching, pushing, straining, and over-taxing your body is a sure way to beat it up. Forget about working through the pain, like the trainers tell you. Don't go there! Pain is Nature's clumsy way of saying "Stop!"

And don't tell me that it's OK for young fit adults. It is NOT. Whatever the trainers tell you, exercise beyond gentle moderation is going to KILL you. Strong language—but I never mince words.

I remember well the story of Joss Naylor, from Cumbria, the English Lake District where I had a cottage for 15 years before coming to the USA. Joss was a local legend. In 1975 he set a record for climbing 72 mountain peaks involving over 100 miles (160 km) and 37,000 feet (11,000 m) of ascent in just under 24 hours (23h20m). It's mind boggling to try to grasp.

But would I envy Joss, his fitness and performance? Not at all. Despite obviously having superb physical fitness and the discipline of mind to carry out exercise at a level, which takes our breath away just to think about it, Joss's body was so brutalized by the age of 50 that he was racked with arthritis (it didn't stop him running but it did stop him from aging successfully).

> **Inappropriate exercise can do more harm than good.**

Inappropriate exercise can do more harm than good, with the definition of "inappropriate" varying according to the individual. For many activities, especially running, there are significant injuries that occur with poorly regimented exercise schedules. In extreme instances, over-exercising induces serious performance loss.

Unaccustomed overexertion of muscles leads to rhabdomyolysis (damage to muscle) most often seen in new army recruits. [Jimenez, C., Pacheco, E., Moreno, A., Carpenter, A. 1996. A Soldier's Neck and Shoulder Pain. The Physician and Sports medicine, 24(6), 81–82. Retrieved October 5, 2006, from ProQuest database].

Excess exercise can also cause loss of periods (amenorrhea) in women. Since preserving our hormone function is critical, this does not seem a logical way to go for keen anti-agers. We don't want periods after the menopause, of course, but we do want some of that residual progesterone and estrogen. It keeps you young!

What I put more emphasis on is quality of movement. To walk along with your body, rejoicing in the rhythm of steps and arm swing, brings a whole lot more to bear on the concept of "wellbeing" than just setting records for work done or physiological output.

Not that you need be shy of exertion, if you like some. There are plenty of accounts of octogenarians (and beyond) running marathons. But I will reserve judgment until we see just how much harm these aging over-achievers cause to themselves!

Eight Scientific Studies Show Why Not To Exercize Hard

Ayurvedic medicine has taught for 7,000 years that excessive exertion is bad. Dr. Li (page 8) who lived to over 250 years of age said be like a tortoise!

Yet Western folly has the motto "No pain, no gain". Well, I have a better saying: "Pain means you are damaging your body and excessive pain may mean permanent damage. So don't do it!"

If you think I'm crazy and way out of step, here are 8 scientific studies that will rock your complacency (compiled by Joe Mercola).

1. According to a study presented at the Canadian Cardiovascular Congress 2010 in Montreal, regular exercise reduces cardiovascular risk by a factor of two or three, but the extended vigorous exercise performed during a marathon raises your cardiac risk seven-fold!

2. In a 2011 study published in the Journal of Applied Physiology, researchers recruited a group of extremely fit older men, all members of the 100 Marathon club (having completed a minimum of 100 marathons). Half of the men showed heart muscle scarring as a result of their endurance running—specifically, the half who had trained the longest and hardest. If running marathons provided cardiovascular benefit, this group would have had the healthiest hearts! [J Appl Physiol. 2011 Jun;110(6):1622-6. doi: 10.1152/japplphysiol.01280.2010. Epub 2011 Feb 17, Diverse patterns of myocardial fibrosis in lifelong, veteran endurance athletes.]

3. A 2011 rat study published in the journal Circulation was designed to mimic the strenuous daily exercise load of serious marathoners over the course of 10 years. All the rats had normal, healthy hearts at the outset of the study, but by the end, most of them had developed "diffuse scarring and some structural changes, similar to the changes seen in the human endurance athletes." [Circulation. 2011; 123: 13-22 Published online before print December 20, 2010, doi: 10.1161]

4. A 2012 study in the European Heart Journal found that long-term endurance athletes suffer from diminished function of the right ventricle of the heart and increased cardiac enzymes (markers for heart injury) after endurance racing, which may activate platelet formation and clotting. Twelve percent of the athletes had detectable scar tissue on their heart muscle one week post-race. [Eur Heart J (2012) 33 (8): 998-1006]

5. A 2010 study presented by the American College of Cardiology showed that endurance runners have more calcified plaque in their arteries (which also increases stroke and dementia risk) than those who are not endurance athletes. [Schwartz JG. Does long-term endurance running enhance or inhibit coronary artery plaque formation? A prospective multidetector CTA study of men completing marathons for at least 25 consecutive years. Presented at: American College of Cardiology 59th Annual Scientific Sessions; March 13-16, 2010; Atlanta]

6. A 2011 German study revealed a very high incidence of carotid and peripheral atherosclerosis among male marathon runners. [Med Sci Sports Exerc. 2011 Jul;43(7):1142-7. doi: 10.1249/MSS.0b013e3182098a51. Carotid and peripheral atherosclerosis in male marathon runners]

7. A 2006 study screened 60 non-elite participants of the 2004 and 2005 Boston Marathons, using echocardiography and serum biomarkers. Researchers found decreased right ventricular systolic function in the runners, caused by an increase in inflammation and a decrease in blood flow. [Circulation. 2006; 114: 2325-2333]

8. Research by Dr. Arthur Siegel, director of Internal Medicine at Harvard's McLean Hospital, also found that long-distance running leads to high levels of inflammation that may trigger cardiac events. [Am J Cardiol. 2001 Oct 15;88(8):918-20, A9. Effect of marathon running on inflammatory and hemostatic markers]

Being a Couch Potato is Bad!

What you need is moderate and frequent exercise. Slobbing out and becoming a couch potato is unquestionably bad for your mind and body. It will rapidly advance the problems of aging, meaning you may live until you are old but you'll feel it too, with poor memory and cognitive function, stiff and slow movements and pains everywhere (call that living?).

In the US alone, a quarter of a million deaths a year are attributable to sedentary lifestyles. So it's not just a matter of discomfort; lack of exercise can kill you! It may surprise you to learn lack of exercise measurably increases the risk for cardiovascular problems, diabetes, and a host of other diseases, including cancer.

> **In the US alone, a quarter of a million deaths a year are attributable to sedentary lifestyles!**

We need regular exercise to stay supple (very important as we age) and to maintain our muscle strength. You won't be having much sex if every time you exert yourself slightly you gasp and get chest pains! Better to keep fit and be able to meet the demands of spontaneous pleasurable activity.

Something else you may not know. Exertion maintains the strength of our bones. If you don't use them, you lose them applies here too. There are only three solidly proven parameters, which prevent or slow deadly osteoporosis, and physical activity is definitely one of the most important.

(See section on osteoporosis at the end of this chapter.)

Do You Have Sitting Disease?

That's the new buzzword for a sedentary lifestyle, which may put your health at risk.

A growing body of research shows that long periods of physical inactivity raise your risk of developing heart disease, diabetes, cancer, and obesity. We were evolved to move, not sit around.

According to James Levine, MD, PhD, professor of medicine at the Mayo Clinic in Rochester, Minnesota, and author of the book Move a Little, Lose a Lot, "The strangest thing in the world is that people spend all day scrunched in a chair. It's a form of physical entrapment."

> **30 minutes of vigorous walking, three to four times a week is a good baseline.**

Levine's book gives a number of simple solutions, without any workout equipment:

Be NEAT! It stands for non-exercise activity thermogenesis: warm up by stretching, turning, and bending. Non-exercise activities include household chores like folding laundry or mowing the lawn, and simple substitutions such as taking the stairs instead of the elevator. None of those activities requires a gym membership, but all of them burn calories. And if we fail to do them, says Levine, we're being robbed of the chance to burn an extra 1,500 to 2,400 calories per day.

Simple examples include:

- A quick walk around the block before your morning shower
- A 30-minute walk at lunch
- A couple of walk-and-talk meetings during the day. Research shows you'll think better pacing when you're talking on the phone
- Taking a 15-minute catch-up walk after work with your partner
- Walking with your children and listening to their music with them
- Doing some active volunteering such as taking a stressed mom's children out for a walk or bringing a meal to an elderly person.

I used to like dancing in the car (not recommended)! I also had a long spell of setting up my computer and keyboard at standing up height. It needs a higher than normal chair. But it means you can spend a lot of "computer time" moving around. Just sit down again when you're tired. Remember, too long of standing periods can make varicose veins worse.

The important thing is to vary standing and sitting as much as you can. Get up and stretch a few times an hour. It'll refresh you mentally, anyway.

Pretend it's 1985 (before dreaded emails), says Levine. Have a question for your co-worker down the hall? Don't shoot him an e-mail; instead walk to his cubicle and ask him face to face. Some companies have instituted email-free Fridays to get employees out of their chairs more often.

Rearrange the office. Help your company encourage its employees to be more physically active without suggesting that they install treadmills at every workstation, Levine says. Start having walk-and-talk meetings rather than conference room meetings. Move trash cans so people have to walk to use them. Relocate water coolers by windows, where people will want to congregate.

If you have a treadmill, set it up for watching TV, and only allow yourself to watch when you're walking. No exercise equipment? March in place or tidy the room while watching.

Finally, get rid of the park-near-the-door mentality. My wife and I laugh at Americans, who fight in the parking lot to get right by the door of the store or mall, to minimize walking. We take pride in parking half across the lot, so we have to walk to go inside. Try it! Forget about ego and outdoing others. Instead focus on gentle exercise and living longer than those slouches.

How Much Is Good?

30 minutes of vigorous walking, three to four times a week is a good baseline. Try to add to that some cardiovascular workout. It's been shown to play a key role in neurogenesis, that's growing new brain cells, That's just what we want to stay sharp mentally.

By cardio, we mean short bursts where you get out of breath, having created a temporary oxygen deficiency. You'll need to keep it going longer if you want the fat burn but that's different. Talk to a trainer if you're that serious! Good cardio activity is sports: running, tennis, swimming, rowing, cycling etc. In short, anything that gets you out of breath.

Resistance training, although I don't like it myself (boring!), has been shown to benefit the brain and mind. Resistance training means the use of dumbbells, springs, medicine balls and the like. Again, consult with an expert if you are keen on this type of exercise.

Remember your own body is resistance when you do pushups, squats and toil up hill.

Combination activities and sports, especially those that develop hand, eye, and brain coordination are best of all. You can actually grow brain tissue. Dr. Daniel G. Amen MD, author of *Magnificent Mind At Any Age* recommends table tennis, for developing fast, coordinated reflexes and using various parts of the brain as you plan and execute shots at very high speed.

Exercise is a much proven way to prevent strokes, heart disease, osteoporosis, senility, diabetes, and just about anything, it's tested against. Take for example, another meta-analysis on stroke prevention from 2003. This study looked specifically at exercise and stroke risk. In this case, the authors looked at the results of 23 different studies that examined the effect of exercise on stroke risk. Here's what they found:

When they compared highly active exercisers on a case-by-case basis to those who did not exercise, they found that the exercisers were a whopping 64% less likely to have a stroke. Even those who exercised only every now and then still showed a reduction in risk of up to 27%.

[Lee CD, Folsom AR, Blair SN. Physical Activity and Stroke Risk A Meta-Analysis. Stroke. 2003;34:2475-2481]

Have You Heard Of Fit And Fat? It's A Myth!
You've probably heard of the notion of being fat but fit, yes? Somebody who is overweight but exercises regularly is better than somebody slim who is lazy and inactive. Right? **Wrong!**

Researchers report in the April 28 2008 issue of *Archives of Internal Medicine* that although physical activity definitely helps improve cardiovascular health, such exercise does not eliminate the negative effects of being overweight.

In other words, weight is more critical than activity.

About half of the women in the study were considered to be of normal weight. A little less than one-third of the women were overweight, and 18% were truly obese. A BMI between 25 and 29 is considered overweight. A BMI of 30 or above is considered obese. Remember, the older BMI measurement (body-mass index) is not as good a measure as hip-to-waist ratio.

34% of the participants were considered physically active, using the US Surgeon General's guidelines.

During about 11 years of follow-up, 948 women developed heart disease. Moreover, the study showed that active women of normal weight had the lowest heart disease risk. Heart disease risk was slightly higher for women of normal weight who were inactive.

Active women who were overweight or obese were more likely to experience heart disease during follow-up than active normal-weight women, but less likely than their inactive counterparts.

The highest heart disease risk was seen among the most inactive, heaviest women. Simply put, eating less will do more for your health and longevity than regular exercise, though both are measurably important.

[SOURCE: Archives of Internal Medicine, April 28, 2008; vol 168: pp 884-890. News release, JAMA/Archives].

Posture

Posture enters into this too. You can tell someone in an advance state of aging, due to their bent over posture. People reduce in height, as they grow older, not so much due to shrinkage of tissues and spine but more to do with the lack of that elasticity and tone of their skeleton. Simply put, they bend over!

Avoiding rounded shoulders is important and especially difficult if, like me, you spend many hours a day at a desk, heaped over a computer.

The trouble is you have to remember to keep straightening up and adjusting your posture. One idea is to try is to get a back brace. When you first start wearing a brace, it can be uncomfortable, due to placing your body in an unfamiliar posture, albeit a healthier one.

The important thing is that the brace acts as a reminder for you to keep your posture straight. Before you know it, you will no longer need the help of the brace, because your muscles automatically know to hold your shoulders back in the proper position. If you get tired toward the end of the day and notice your shoulders starting to slouch, you can put the brace on for a little extra support.

Take a look here: http://www.gaiam.com/product/wellness-clinic/pain-relief-back-care/view+all/lite+weight+shoulders+back.do?search=basic&keyword=shoulders&sortby=bestSellers&page=1

Sitting on balance balls or backless chairs that support you at the knees can be good too.

Alexander Technique

This is something I really recommend. It does far more than a brace could.

F. Matthias Alexander (1869-1955) was an Australian actor who began to experience chronic laryngitis whenever he performed. When his doctors could not help him, Alexander discovered a solution on his own. He had not been aware that excess tension in his neck and body were causing his problems, and began to find new ways to speak and move with greater ease. He worked on changing his posture.

His health improved to such an extent that his friends and several of the doctors he had consulted earlier persuaded him to teach others what he had learned. Over a career span of more than fifty years, he refined his method of instruction. After teaching for over 35 years, he began to train teachers in what has now become known as the Alexander Technique.

The Alexander Technique is a method that works to change (movement) habits in our everyday activities. It is a simple and practical method for improving ease and freedom of movement, balance, support, and coordination. The technique teaches the use of the appropriate amount of effort for a particular activity, giving you more energy for all your activities.

It is not a series of treatments or exercises, but rather a reeducation of the mind and body. The Alexander Technique is a method, which helps a person discover a new balance in the body, by releasing unnecessary tension. It can be applied to sitting, lying down, standing, walking, lifting, and other daily activities...

You really need an Alexander teacher, although there will always be claims for success with self-taught material.

Alexander, was his own teacher and was fond of remarking, "Anyone can do what I did, IF they will do what I did." But by the end of his life, Alexander had come to the conclusion that attempts to put his teaching into practice without the help of a teacher were often not successful.

Find an Alexander teacher here: http://www.alexandertechnique.com/teacher/

Dance

I think dance has powerful additional factors, over and above the mere expenditure of calories.

When you dance, you feel enlivened, engaged, graceful, and light. Spending energy on dance seems to create more energy. My mother taught dance until she was in her 70s and still dances regularly, despite a stroke, even though the big 90 is coming up soon! I'm sure it keeps her going.

Dance is good for coordination. As I hinted, it makes you feel beautiful, and that's no bad thing at any age.

Music and rhythm is its own thing and very powerful. Its roots go right back to the dawn of our ancestry and is a powerful mind and mood changer. There are many papers showing the important health benefits of music.

It has to be the right music. Hard rock and heavy metal dehydrates and kills plants, so it can't be much good for us. Lively bright music uplifts; solemn music can bring us to rejoicing. It can help out cognitive functions too; I'm sure you've heard of the controversial "Mozart Effect".

Once again, there is surprising science for this "outside the box" idea. In fact clinical studies have shown:

Dance/movement therapy can be effective in …"developing body image, improving self-concept and increasing self-esteem; facilitating attention; ameliorating depression, decreasing fears and anxieties, and expressing anger; decreasing isolation, increasing communication skill, and fostering solidarity; decreasing bodily tension, reducing chronic pain, and enhancing circulatory and respiratory functions; reducing suicidal ideas, increasing feelings of well-being, and promoting healing; and increasing verbalization." [That's verbatim from a report to the US National Institutes of Health on Alternative Systems and Practises, prepared under the auspices of the Workshop on Alternative Medicine, Chantilly, VA September 14- 16, 1992]

Now you know why I am promoting this.

Yoga

Then there is yoga, of course. Unless you have lived on the Planet Zod for the last 50 years, you will have heard of the anti-aging benefits of yoga. Some people swear by it. It's very engaging and has scads of benefits, over and above making you supple. Let's look at some of those benefits.

The Benefits of Yoga

- Yoga cleanses the body and is very effective in a variety of conditions and disorders. There is even yoga therapy available.

- Yoga helps to make you very flexible, having a positive effect on your body's joints, including joints that have been previously injured.

- Lubricates tendons, and ligaments helping to keep your body younger.

- Massages the organs of the body. In fact, it's likely the only activity to do that. This massage and stimulation helps to keep disease away and keep you younger than your actual age.

- Yoga detoxifies the body. When you stretch your muscles and massage your organs there is an increased blood flow, which helps to move toxins out of the body.

- Relaxation is an important component of yoga allowing you to clear the mind and re-energize yourself.

Tai Chi & Qigong

Tai Chi and Qigong, two Chinese wellness practices, have been previously associated with a variety of physical and mental health benefits. Linda Larkey, of Arizona State University (Arizona, USA), and colleagues conducted a meta-analysis of 77 peer-reviewed journal articles that reported on the results of Tai Chi and Qigong interventions.

Assessing data on the 6,410 men and women involved in the 77 studies, the team found that subjects were significantly improved on the health parameters of cardiopulmonary fitness, immune function, bone density, and quality of life, as compared to sedentary counterparts.

The researchers write that: "Research has demonstrated consistent, significant results for a number of health benefits in [clinical trials], evidencing progress toward recognizing the similarity and equivalence of Qigong and Tai Chi."

[Roger Jahnke, Linda Larkey, Carol Rogers, Jennifer Etnier, Fang Lin. "A Comprehensive Review of Health Benefits of Qigong and Tai Chi." American Journal of Health Promotion, July/August 2010, V24, I6, e1-25].

Copied from *worldhealth.net*

Exercise Sleep Crossover

I have emphasized the importance of sound sleep in slowing down aging. There is no question that exercise helps you sleep more soundly and with more benefits. Routine exercise helps normalize melatonin production and so improves sleeping habits. You only have to think back to the last time you had a long, physically active day, then slumped on the sofa, and fell asleep in minutes to know this is true!

Some people suffer sleep deprivation due to waking too early in the morning. This is one of the classic signs of depression. If you experience regular early morning waking, get to work on the brain nourishment chapter and fix it (only very rarely is depression a matter for an MD, it's so easy to self-regulate).

Exercise causes the release of endorphins into the body. These endorphins create a feeling of well-being, even euphoria. This is an excellent means of combating depression and getting a good night's sleep.

Exercise also helps to release much-needed serotonin into the body. Serotonin helps in regulating sleep patterns. That is, it kind of regulates your internal clock. It also helps in combating depression, as well as many forms of mental illness.

In general, however, I agree with the consensus that exertion just before going to bed will tend to keep you awake.

Only in cases of extreme insomnia, would I prescribe the following sleep remedy, rather than resort to drugs or even herbs. Try allocating an evening workout session if you really suffer badly with insomnia, as follows:

- After you evening meal, go for a walk. Walk away from the house until you are really tired.

- Then turn around and walk back. Then you will be even more tired. You should sleep soundly.

A combination of exercise and sound sleep can leave you feeling energized and looking better, which may have a positive effect on your sex life. Regular physical activity can lead to enhanced arousal for women, and men who exercise regularly are less likely to have problems with erectile dysfunction than are men who don't exercise — especially as they get older.

Osteoporosis and Bone Strength

This critical factor to be avoided in successful aging is often ignored. Hormones and super nutrients may be more glamorous. Nearly a third of all American women will develop osteoporosis during their lifetime and it will be severe enough to cause a fracture. In fact, at least 1.2 million fractures are said to occur each year as a direct result of this condition. Do I have your attention now?

The medical and social costs of osteoporosis are estimated to be from $6 billion to upwards of $10 billion annually. It affects 15 to 20 million Americans (mostly women) annually, and each year there are 200,000 hip fractures attributed to osteoporosis.

We should not forget that the complications of a hip fracture are fatal to many of these patients. In fact, more women die every year of hip fracture than all those who die of cancer of the breast, cervix or uterus combined. The UK picture is equally gloomy.

Hormone Therapy

The current therapy focuses mainly on estrogen, supposedly to retard the advance of the menopause, and calcium supplementation, since osteoporosis is seen largely as a loss of calcium tissue in the bones. However, it is probably not really as simple as this.

Estrogen therapy really only defers the inevitable and therefore its 'success' as a treatment is debatable. Moreover, some doctors would see the risk of hormone replacement therapy as wholly unacceptable when used for this purely prophylactic reason.

Calcium supplements (around 800 to 1500 mg a day) are usually recommended but it must be said that studies on how effective this is are confused and contradictory. Calcium supplementation will not restore lost bone tissue. The likelihood is that calcium supplementation is of little value on its own.

The paradox is that it is known that calcium deposition is a factor in hardening of the arteries, arthritis, kidney stones, gallstones, and cataracts, so for some patients it may be a question of aging one way or decaying another.

In my view (based on over 40 years clinical experience), osteoporosis is best seen as a systemic nutritional disease. Just topping up with calcium is a waste of time unless the causes of bone

Dr. Keith special insights

First, FORGET CALCIUM. Calcium deficiency is not the cause of osteoporosis. In fact calcium is the last thing we need as we age: calcium deposits are what cause arthritic joints, deafness, brain aging and hardening of the arteries. Today, one of the number one markers for heart attack and death is measurable deposits of calcium in the coronary arteries and nearby aorta.

As I said, who needs calcium?

Magnesium and boron are what we really want. Let's get at the real story...

Formerly known as senile osteoporosis, it is now obvious that in women the bone mass begins to decline even before menopause, at around 35 years of age, and then accelerates rapidly for some eight to ten years. Thereafter it continues at a slower rate.

It is a disease of Western women. Chinese female octogenarians, for example, show almost no osteoporosis or fractures of the femur. This leads to the speculation that osteoporosis is an environmental condition, caused mainly by diet.

depletion are addressed. Bisphophonate drugs are a very stupid approach and should never, ever be considered, since they wreak healthy metabolism.

Bone Densitometry

Probably the single biggest factor in whether a woman will develop osteoporosis is her bone density at the age of 35. Those with dense bones are unlikely to reach severe osteoporotic levels even during the seventh and eight decade. Those whose bones are thin even before menopause are likely to end up with difficulties, no matter what treatment is attempted. It is to be hoped that routine bone densitometry screening will be available to all menopausal women.

> **Those with dense bones are unlikely to reach severe osteoporotic levels even during the seventh and eight decade.**

The truth is that osteoporosis is probably a holistic condition and needs treating holistically. It is doubtful if single nutrient supplements, even such obvious ones as calcium and vitamin D, would be effective in the absence of good whole-body nutrition.

Bone, remember, is more than just a collection of calcium apatite crystals. It is an active living tissue, constantly remodeling itself through deposition and absorption and continually participating in a wide range of biochemical reactions — reactions that will be compromised by any degree of under nutrition.

Nutritional Factors Affecting Bone Strength

Vitamin K is known to be important primarily for its effects on blood clotting. However, it is also required for synthesizing osteocalcin, a protein found uniquely in bone and on which the calcium crystallizes. It is usually assumed that vitamin K deficiency is rare, but in one study (of only 16 patients) with osteoporosis, their mean serum vitamin K levels were only 35% of those of age-matched controls.

Vitamin D is required for intestinal calcium absorption. Reduced vitamin D levels are common in elderly patients, especially women. Studies have failed to show conclusively that vitamin D supplements help, yet it would be logical to ensure that D status is adequate.

Magnesium

Magnesium is probably far more important than calcium, but scientific proof is lacking. The critical bone enzyme *alkaline phosphatase* (involved in forming new calcium crystals) is activated by magnesium.

Its relative lack, therefore, could be expected to block the deposition of new bone tissue. Whole-body concentrations of magnesium were found to be below normal in 16 out of 19 osteoporotic women.

Manganese is also required for bone mineralization. Rats fed on manganese-deficient diets had smaller and less dense bones. In one study of osteoporotic women, blood manganese levels were found to be only 25 per cent of those of controls! About 5 mg daily is accepted generally as a suitable supplement.

Folic Acid

The interest in this vitamin co-factor stems from the fact that homocystine metabolism seems to be at least partially folic acid-dependent, and patients with a genetic failure in the metabolism of homocystine are known to develop severe osteoporosis at an early age. Folic acid deficiency is relatively common, particularly in those who do not follow a hunter-gatherer type diet. Supplementation would therefore seem to be prudent.

Boron

Previously thought to be important only for plants, we now know that boron plays a role in human nutrition, particularly in relation to bone health. Supplementing the diet with boron (3 mg daily) was shown to reduce urinary calcium excretion by 44%. Interestingly, it also increased the serum concentration of the hormone 17-beta-oestradiol, which may be the most biologically active form of naturally occurring human estrogen. Dietary requirements are not known; supplementation is suggested at 2 to 3 mg per day.

Strontium

Strontium has been shown to prevent chemical irritations of the skin, it plays an important role in building strong bones, reduces dental cavities, and bone pain.

In the largest published clinical trial, 1,649 postmenopausal women with osteoporosis received 680 mg per day of strontium or placebo for three years. Compared to the placebo group, strontium reduced the incidence of vertebral fractures by 49% in just one year.

We used to get adequate strontium through our drinking water, and through foods since it is naturally present in water and soil. However, these days it's almost impossible to get strontium this way because of water treatment that kills strontium and soil that has lost all of its nutritional value because of overuse.

According to one study, 170 mg of strontium per day, seems to be more effective than 680 mg per day for reducing fracture risk, which raises the question as to whether a lower dose might be as effective.

Other Important Nutrients

Attention has also been focused on a number of other nutrients including silicon, vitamin B6, zinc, copper, and vitamin C. In other words, we are working towards the conclusion that any important nutrient could lead to as yet undiscovered deficiencies in bone metabolism; good holistic nutrition is vital.

Non-Nutritional Factors
- Exercise has been shown to have a positive effect on bone density; thus, those who lead sedentary lives are more likely to develop osteoporosis. Animal studies show that lack of use leads to rapid bone re-absorption (breakdown by cells). Therefore, it is likely regular gentle exercise will benefit all women at or beyond the menopausal years.

- Some drugs accelerate bone loss. Particularly important are steroids such as prednisolone, though it appears that the type of osteoporosis this can lead to is quite different biochemically from post-menopausal osteoporosis. Certain anticonvulsants (phenytoin, for example) may also lead to increased bone reabsorption.

- Smoking is said to hasten the menopause by about five years and reduces oestrogen levels thereafter. Other evidence suggests that smoking may alter osteoblast function (osteoblasts are the cells that 'build' bone).

- There are also racial and genetic factors.

In any clinical evaluation of osteoporosis, a number of disease states need to be considered. All are rightly the preserve of a qualified physician, and are not for self--medication. They include anorexia nervosa, testicular failure, thyrotoxicosis, bone cancer disease, and immobilization after surgery.

14 | Miscellaneous Factors

Here I have grouped together a series of relevant anti-aging factors, which don't easily fit elsewhere. But do remember all aspects of anti-aging are inter-related. Diet is connected with inflammation, carbohydrate control, arterial health, good brain function; lack of stress and sound sleep is associated with hormone balance, better heart rate variability, and so forth.

Fundamental health principle: all disease phenomena are caused by a complex cascade of failures. There is no "one cause" of disease. Even tuberculosis is not "caused" by the TB bacterium (*Mycobacterium tuberculosis*); it's caused by malnutrition, leading to a poor immune system, usually coupled with a romantic shock (actually proven by science!) AND the opportune presence of Mycobacterium tuberculosis.

All body systems and functions interconnect and depend on each other. It is the height of medical folly to have an oncologist who couldn't recognize a nutritional deficiency if it kicked him; or a psychiatrist who didn't look for organ disease; or a dermatologist who couldn't see the patient was pregnant! But it happens… a lot!

I just prefer to lay out these additional elements here, rather than let any one chapter get too overloaded.

Sleep and Vitality

Get adequate sleep! A team of British and Italian researchers found people who sleep less than six hours a night are 12% more likely to die prematurely than those who get the recommended six to eight hours of slumber, a new study has found.

Unfortunately, it doesn't cut the other way. Sleep longer than 8 hours doesn't increase your life span! More than nine hours a night might be an important sign of a serious or potentially fatal illness.

The researchers reviewed 16 studies that included more than 1.3 million people who were followed for up to 25 years. In that time, more than 100,000 deaths were recorded among the participants, who were from Asia, Europe and the United States.

The findings provide unequivocal evidence of the direct link between insufficient sleep and increased risk of premature death, said the authors of the study, which is published in the May 2010 issue of Sleep.

According to Francesco Cappuccio, leader of the Sleep, Health and Society Program at the University of Warwick in the United Kingdom, lack of sleep should be regarded as a behavioral risk factor, or risk marker, for disease and early death. "Consistently sleeping six to eight hours per night may be optimal for health," he concluded.

> **People who sleep less than six hours a night are 12% more likely to die prematurely.**

Inadequate or broken sleep, just a few hours a night, can hinder metabolism and hormone production in a way that is similar to the effects of aging and the early stages of diabetes. Chronic sleep loss may speed the onset or increase the severity of age-related conditions such as type 2 diabetes, high blood pressure, obesity, and memory loss. The researchers showed that just one week of sleep deprivation seriously altered subject's hormone levels and their capacity to metabolize carbohydrates. People who trade sleep for work or play may get used to it and feel less fatigued but there is always a pay-off.

During sleep-deprivation testing, researchers found the subject's blood sugar levels took 40% longer to drop following a high-carbohydrate meal, compared with the sleep-recovery period. Their ability to secrete and respond to the hormone insulin, which helps regulate blood sugar, dropped by 30%.

This is what happens when an individual develops insulin resistance, a precursor to type 2 diabetes. In addition, the sleep-deprived subjects had higher nighttime concentrations of the hormone cortisol, which also helps regulate blood sugar, and lower levels of thyroid-stimulating hormone. These raised cortisol levels mimic levels that are often seen in older people, and may be involved in age-related insulin resistance and memory loss. [The Lancet October 23, 1999;354:1435-1439].

Just to confirm that suspicion, another important study published in the June 2010 issue of the Journal of Clinical Endocrinology & Metabolism showed that even missing *just one night's sleep* does increase insulin resistance. It is NOT a fixed factor.

The study included nine healthy people whose insulin sensitivity was measured after a night of normal sleep (about eight hours) and after a night of four hours of sleep.

"Our data indicate that insulin sensitivity is not fixed in healthy subjects, but depends on the duration of sleep in the preceding night," lead author Dr. Esther Donga, of the Leiden University Medical Center in the Netherlands, said in a news release from The Endocrine Society. "In fact, it is tempting to speculate that the negative effects of multiple nights of shortened sleep on glucose tolerance can be reproduced, at least in part, by just one sleepless night."

It's interesting that sleep duration, on the whole, has shortened considerably in western societies in the past decade. This coincides with a marked rise in the incidence of type 2 diabetes.

Is There A Causative Link?
The study findings make it clear that sleep deprivation has more profound effects on metabolic regulation than previously appreciated.

Sleep debts are sort of like stress. Cortisol levels drop with adequate sleep. Most sleep-deprivation research has focused on what it does to the brain, but it is likely that sleep has many functions. In the study, subjects' blood sugar and hormone concentrations were restored after the sleep-recovery period.

Earlier research has shown that in developed countries, the average night's sleep has grown shorter since the beginning of the century, from 9 hours to 7.5 hours. Many people give up sleep to make room for work and leisure. An adequate amount of sleep is as important as an adequate amount of exercise. Sleeping is not a waste of time; sleeping will give you back years at the end of your life!

Remedy
Don't forget to try the sleep dep remedy on page 175.

Coffee an Anti-Ager?
Drinking coffee may extend life; who'd have thought it?

We have to be cautious with this but it does seem like good news for some. I've been following the literature for years and have noticed studies showing that coffee helps diminish the risk of a number of conditions, including Alzheimer's, cardiovascular disease, diabetes, Parkinson's disease and colon cancer.

Now new research suggests that drinking coffee, even in large amounts, might help you live longer. It wasn't a big difference mind you - not enough to suggest everyone should drink coffee. Also, it didn't make any difference whether you drank decaf or not.

But it might be telling us that coffee isn't actually harmful.

Among women, drinking two to three cups of coffee a day was associated with an 18% reduction in death from all causes, while drinking four to five cups was associated with a 26% reduction in risk.

The risk reduction in men was smaller and could have been due to chance.

My own take on this, entirely independently of the study (but based on decades of clinical experience), is that ground coffee is much healthier. When making espresso or percolating coffee we get only the aqueous extract of flavors and incidental substances. With instant coffee the whole bean is ground up and we end up swallowing many complex resinous and insoluble residues. Some of these, I'm sure, are not good for us.

Anti-Inflammatory?

It has been suggested that coffee may protect against heart disease and other aging processes by reducing inflammation. Coffee has also been shown to lower blood sugar levels, which could have a beneficial effect on diabetes risk.

Coffee supplies beneficial plant antioxidants known as polyphenols. For those who eat mainly junk this could be their main source of these important dietary nutrients.

It was a good study, with solid design. No flaws. Just remember that the schlock you put with coffee (cream etc) is what's really deadly for your health!

> [Lopez-Garcia, E., Annals of Internal Medicine, June 17, 2008; vol 48: pp 904-915. Ester Lopez-Garcia, PhD, department of preventive medicine and public health, University of Madrid, Madrid, Spain.]

And another study in relation to deadly oral cancers:

University of Milan researchers Carlotta Galeone, ScD, PhD, and colleagues compared 5,139 people with head and neck cancer to 9,028 people without cancer. They found that people who drink more than four cups of coffee each day have 39% lower odds of getting mouth or throat cancer than people who don't drink coffee. That's rather striking! The protection didn't hold up for cancer of the larynx though.

Drinking less than five cups of coffee a day had a smaller but still statistically significant protective effect: about 4% lower odds of mouth and throat cancer for each cup drunk daily.

> [Galeone, C. Cancer Epidemiology, Biomarkers, & Prevention, July 2010]

Just remember this was a European study. Coffee from Starbucks is not the same! It's filled with schlock and disgusting calories. You need espresso or Americano (black) to match these results.

Hmmm. That Dreamy Smell…

Maybe we don't even need to drink the coffee to get some benefits! We assume that the wake up taste and the caffeine shock are what coffee is all about. But wait a minute… What if merely waking up and smelling coffee powers up your brain, without ever taking a sip?

New research published in the *Journal of Agricultural and Food Chemistry*, June 25th, 2008, is shedding light on how drinking and smelling coffee might affect genes and proteins in the brain. The study, led by Han-Seouk Seo of Seoul National University, is probably the first research to look at how just the aroma of coffee affects us, or at least how it affects lab rats, some of which were sleep deprived.

The rats (poor things) were first stressed up with lack of sleep and then exposed to coffee bean aroma. Well it sounds cruel, until you consider what geeks and nerds do to themselves in the small hours of the night!

Seo and colleagues found that coffee-sniffing, sleep-deprived rats showed different levels of activity in 17 genes in the brain. This is almost incredible. The researchers also found the just the aroma changed the levels of some brain proteins in ways that could have a calming effect on stress or have antioxidant function.

There is the usual problem, of course: does this translate directly to humans?

Well folks, you can join the scientific community. Get yourself a bag of roasted coffee beans near your desk for that four o'clock slump and see if taking a whiff will perk you up!

All I know is that just to smell it is as good as to drink it and, in some cases, the smell is better than the resultant bitter brew (I only drink strong decaf espresso, without sugar or sweetener).

Let me know what you find!

Enjoy a Glass of Red Wine!

So what about alcohol? Is it good after all?

Let's start by straightening out the confusion. You'll read reports that say alcohol will enable you to live longer and you should drink some; other reports say it's bad and you shouldn't drink any; then yet other reports (which make me laugh) prove alcohol is good for you but then say you shouldn't drink any way!

A lot of social prejudice and "party line" thinking gets in the way of true science. Researchers seem to worry that people will think them irresponsible if they hold to what they proved, that alcohol in certain forms can be beneficial.

These are the facts in a nutshell; from these you can "interpret" what you read and hear.

1. Alcohol in excess in all forms is bad for you. It is associated with heart disease, cancer and a host of avoidable pathology. There is no question that alcohol in excess causes dyslipidemia of the blood (wrong fats) and can of course lead to cirrhosis.

2. Excess is an almost unquantifiable variable. Some people can drink a bottle of wine a day and feel no ill effect (me for instance!) Others feel bad after a glass. But I can say that generally all alcohol studies are flawed by the fact that people lie about what they drink (except me!)

    So when you see studies showing that a certain levels of alcohol indulgence produce a certain health change, it almost certainly means a gross *underestimate* of the quantities that cause harm. In other words, it far safer than they claim.

3. Statistics about alcohol-related deaths include stupid things like road traffic accidents, which have nothing to do with the health effects of alcohol. It's false reporting.

4. Moderate alcohol intake of all kinds may have key health benefits, notably reducing stress and increasing the feeling of relaxation, friendship, love and belonging—all of which spin can off hidden benefits.

5. The definitions of moderate vary according to scientists. The idea of 2 small glasses being "moderate" is nonsense. 3 large glasses for a man is moderate (refer to item 2).

6. Most studies showing physiological and anti-aging benefits are based around wine.

7. Most studies condemning "alcohol" lump together beer, spirits and wines. The dangers of spirits cancels out the well-proven benefits of wine.

8. So it comes down to this: wine drinking is probably good in moderation. The so-called "French paradox" is about the fact that most French people drink LARGE amounts of wine a day and yet do not suffer worse health as a consequence; they do not die younger as the anti-alcohol brigade tell you they must.

9. Teetotallers don't live as long as moderate drinkers. So no alcohol is not a good option!

10. Alcoholism is a psychological disease as much as an addiction. The person drinks because of stress and pain. The problem is not the alcohol, the problem is the person's life and surroundings.

Just to complete that picture, light drinkers live 2 years longer than average and heavy drinkers (more than 4 drinks a day) live 5-10 years less. Of course, it depends how much they drink, as well as on metabolic differences that enable some individuals to metabolize alcohol faster than others. There are currently no known drugs or other ingestible agents which will accelerate alcohol breakdown. Alcohol ingestion can be slowed by ingesting alcohol on a full stomach. Alcohol is absorbed more rapidly from carbonated drinks, which is bad news for champagne lovers.

Defining Drinking Levels

Here is a refreshingly honest study from Brazil, in the April 2010 issue of the journal *Alcoholism: Clinical & Experimental Research*, which didn't try to bend the findings to fit pre-existing prejudice:

It showed that one or two alcoholic drinks a day may help older people stay mentally sharp.

Researchers asked people 60 and older about their use of alcohol and tested them for dementia and other age-related mental impairments. Not surprisingly, heavy alcohol drinkers had higher rates of mental decline and dementia than elderly teetotalers. But mild to moderate alcohol consumption appeared to be protective.

Here's the point: for the purposes of the study, heavy alcohol use was defined as drinking 2 ounces of ethanol or more a day for men and 1 ounce of ethanol a day for women.

A 5-ounce glass of wine, a 12-ounce glass of regular beer, and a cocktail with 1 1/2 ounces of 80-proof liquor all have about 0.6 ounces of ethanol. So for a man, 3 glasses of wine, 3 beers or 3 shots all score as "moderate" (a bit more liberal than many studies, I may say).

Overall, about 8% of the study participants reported heavy alcohol use, including 17% of males and 3% of females. Heavy means MORE than 3 drinks a day.

In addition:

- A total of 42% of study participants drank alcohol but were not considered heavy drinkers, including 51% of males and 37% of females.

- As a group, mild to moderate alcohol users were more highly educated and better off economically, than non-drinkers.

- About 19% of participants showed some evidence of cognitive and functional impairment and 6% were considered to have dementia.

- Heavy alcohol use was found to be associated with more mental decline and dementia, especially in women, when compared to people who did not drink alcohol at all.

Of course this publication is accompanied by the usual party line rhetoric: "Can't recommend alcohol etc..." Why not, if your science is any good? I recommend wine highly (in moderation, naturally) as a great way to ease stress and enrich our lives with camaraderie. As the Italian's say "A day without wine is a day without sunshine".

Just don't overdo it, OK? (Drinking with food is safest, this is rarely factored in by research studies.)

Resveratrol
A study published in the prestigious journal *Nature* (01 Nov 2006) has shown that resveratrol, an antioxidant found in red wine, extended survival rates of mice and prevented weight-gain from high-calorie diets.

In this study, described by an independent expert (and presumably a wine drinker!) as potentially "the breakthrough of the year", resveratrol consumption was shown to bring a wide range of health benefits, including brain and mental health, and cardiovascular health.

The mice also showed increased insulin sensitivity and decreased glucose levels (counters to diabetes). According to one of the study authors David Sinclair from Harvard Medical School, these positive clinical indicators may mean we can stave off in humans age-related diseases such as type 2 diabetes, heart disease, and cancer, "But only time and more research will tell."

When the study mice reached 'old age' (114 weeks), lead author Joseph Baur and his colleagues report that more than 50 per cent of the high calorie mice had died compared to less than 33 per cent of the high calorie mice receiving resveratrol.

"After six months, resveratrol essentially prevented most of the negative effects of the high calorie diet," said Rafael de Cabo, Ph.D., from the National Institute on Aging (NIA).

"This study shows that an orally available small molecule at doses achievable in humans can safely reduce many of the negative consequences of excess caloric intake, with an overall improvement in health and survival," concluded the researchers.

While the results are very promising, Richard Hodes, M.D., director of the NIA, added a note of perspective and caution: "At the same time, it should be cautioned that this is a study of male mice, and we still have much to learn about resveratrol's safety and effectiveness in humans."

Professor Steve Bloom, an obesity researcher at Imperial College, London, told the BBC: "This paper is extremely interesting - it could be the breakthrough of the year, with massive possibilities for... human beings."

By all means have a glass, if it doesn't give you migraines. But before you change to a French-style 4-hour meal with 2 bottles of wine apiece, be warned: the amount of resveratrol in a glass of red wine is only 0.3 per cent of the relative resveratrol dose given to the gluttonous mice!

The amount of resveratrol in a bottle of red wine can vary between types of grapes and growing seasons, and can vary between 0.2 and 5.8 milligrams per liter. Nearly all dark red wines - merlot, cabernet, zinfandel, shiraz and pinot noir - contain resveratrol.

The study was funded in part by the National Institute on Aging (NIA) of the National Institutes of Health (NIH).

The Real Demon in Drink
The real danger of alcohol is not ethanol itself but a breakdown product (metabolite) called *acetaldehyde*. It's quite poisonous and has been studied extensively. Some recent research is definitely worth sharing here.

We talk of detox pathways in the liver, but remember I told you (page 77) that this is the wrong expression: biotransformation is the correct term. What happens in the liver certainly alters a poison but does not always detoxify it. In fact the change could make it even more poisonous.

That's exactly what happens to alcohol. It's poisonous enough in large doses. But then it is transformed by 6 enzymes called alcohol dehydrogenase (because it takes off the hydrogen, silly!) This turns it into acetaldehyde, a substance capable of giving you a vicious headache and making you vomit.

Acetaldehyde is a powerful muscle poison, roughly 30 times more toxic than ethanol itself. It has been suggested that acetaldehyde is the real demon in the demon drink!

For 30 years researchers have known that excessive alcohol intake causes serious long-term damage to virtually every internal organ: brain, kidneys, gonads, skeletal muscle, liver, heart, uterus and digestive system.

The assumption was that ethanol itself was to blame, but the mechanism was unclear. Now, as we find out more about how drink wreaks long-term havoc, the spotlight is increasingly moving away from ethanol and towards acetaldehyde.

Alcohol may be relatively blameless. Now wouldn't that be an irony!

Our basic diet contains sources of deadly acetaldehyde. Anything fermented will contain some aldehydes: from pickles and yogurts to bread and cheese. Acetaldehyde also occurs naturally in ripe fruit and coffee. Acetaldehyde may be used to produce a deliberate fruity taste. Some yoghurt producers are searching for new bacteria that are even better acetaldehyde producers!

A Few Figures

The average liver processes about 7 grams of ethanol an hour meaning that it takes about 12 hours to eliminate all the ethanol in a bottle of wine. Heavy drinkers generate more alcohol dehydrogenase for themselves and so can do better, say clearing it in 6-8 hours. Until it is gone, we are continuously exposed to acetaldehyde, which follows in its wake.

What is becoming increasingly clear is that almost any exposure to acetaldehyde can do serious damage. Acetaldehyde attaches itself to amino groups in proteins to form stable compounds called adducts which can cause irreversible damage by messing up protein structure and function. After a heavy drinking session, a whole range of adducts are formed in the liver, muscles, heart, brain and gastrointestinal tract.

Skeletal muscle is particularly badly affected and rats given a single dose of ethanol end up with significant muscle damage as a result of acetaldehyde attacking proteins. This means that our traditional view – that mainly the liver and brain gets damaged by drink – is actually incorrect.

> **The average liver processes about 7 grams of ethanol an hour meaning that it takes about 12 hours to eliminate all the ethanol in a bottle of wine.**

The picture is complicated by the fact that the immune system gets drawn in. Adducts are seen as foreign protein and sets off a whole inflammatory response. This is confirmed by the fact that 70% of patients with alcoholic liver disease have anti-acetaldehyde antibodies in their bloodstream. Inflammation is bad in all circumstances except infection. As we have seen earlier, it is the basis of almost all aging and degenerative diseases, from cancer to Alzheimer's, diabetes to arteriosclerosis (New Scientist, 22 May 2004, p 40).

Acetaldehyde also attacks DNA. In 2005, researchers at the US National Institute on Alcohol Abuse and Alcoholism in Bethesda, Maryland, reported that acetaldehyde can attack DNA in much the same way it does proteins. The resulting adducts disrupt DNA's structure and function, and can trigger mutations and chromosomal problems. Not surprisingly then, acetaldehyde is implicated as a carcinogen.

You will have read that alcohol and cancer is linked, especially cancer of the mouth and digestive tract.

In heavy drinkers who lack the breakdown enzyme for acetaldehyde, we observe the incidence of upper gastrointestinal tract cancer is about 50 times the normal rate. It was a cause of great sadness to TV fans around the world that actor John Thaw (Inspector Morse) departed this life too soon. He had esophageal cancer and there is little doubt that this was related to his heavy drinking habits.

A 1998 study of 818 heavy drinkers in Germany found that those individuals who were exposed to excess acetaldehyde as a result of a genetic defect were at greater risk of developing cancers of the upper gastrointestinal tract and liver (International Journal of Cancer, vol 118, p 1998). There are many similar findings that steer towards an inevitable conclusion: that acetaldehyde is a human carcinogen.

Acetaldehyde may also play a role in breast cancer, with up to 5% of all breast cancers attributable to alcohol consumption. The rising rates of liver, colon and rectal cancer in the West may be linked to steadily rising alcohol intake. But again, acetaldehyde and the tricky genes which slow the breakdown process may be the real culprits.

There are even suggestions of a link between acetaldehyde and Alzheimer's disease. In 2004, researchers at Nippon Medical School in Kawasaki, Japan, reported that among a group of people with Alzheimer's, the faulty version of the enzyme gene was significantly more common than among a randomly chosen group of healthy people of the same age (Annals of the New York Academy of Sciences, vol 1011, p 36).

Caution
So this news should instill a certain sense of caution among drinkers. If you are a slow metabolizer, you should drink little or not at all. That much is clear.

But how would you know? If you really care, get yourself a consumer breathalyzer from somewhere like www.breathalyzer.net and practice using it. The actual blood levels are not as significant as how fast they fall off, after your last drink.

To repeat: even low levels of alcohol intake can be dangerous to slow metabolizers. The steady accumulation of acetaldehyde is what is dangerous.

Do remember that a number of alcoholic drinks contain acetaldehyde by intention. Sherry producers, for instance, encourage acetaldehyde production for its fruity aroma. The deeply aromatic flavors of brandy come from a complex mixture of various alcohols, so-called congeners, and acetaldehyde. Calvados (aka. applejack) is particularly rich in acetaldehyde, and it may be significant that regular calvados drinkers have twice the incidence of esophageal and oral cancer compared with wine drinkers who consume the same amount of alcohol.

The Dangers in Your Mouth

Everyone knows that you can tell the age and condition of a horse from its teeth. It should come as no surprise therefore to know that there is a strong connection between human teeth and aging. History tells us that at the start of the twentieth century, one of the single biggest risk factors for early death was in the mouth (infected teeth sending bacterial abscesses to the brain, heart and other organs; in the days before antibiotics, this was deadly).

Surprisingly, at the end of the twentieth century, the picture was remarkably similar. Not exactly teeth, but periodontal (gum) disease had emerged as one of the outstanding markers for risk of serious or fatal heart disease, according to latest research.

As top UK holistic dentist John Roberts points out, most people have a mouth, which contains considerable "open" infection that is putting our internal tissues directly in contact with the outside world. This is not recognized because the septic plaques are hidden under the gum margins and deep within the jaw bone. It poses a serious threat, even in this day and age of antibiotics.

People still die of a tooth abscess. Part of the problem is that the teeth sockets are deep within the skull and very close to the brain. Remarkable x-rays taken at the Karoliska Institute in Stockholm show that infected matter from the jaws and teeth can travel backwards, through interconnecting veins, directly into the brain and ménages. But infected matter can access the bloodstream and end up almost anywhere in the body, to our great peril.

We are far too complacent with this health and aging hazard. You must look after your teeth and gums far better. Now research has directly connected the number of teeth lost with the risk of catastrophic heart disease. As the table shows, the more teeth lost, the greater the risk.

Dental hygiene

Get your oral hygiene in shape, **HOWEVER** (note the emphasis) you need to know that the time when you visit the dentist or even just having the hygienist messing with the de-scaler on your gum margin is the time when torrents of bacteria are disturbed and unleashed into the bloodstream. This is the most dangerous moment. In the old days—and I'm old enough to talk about the old days—people at risk of serious heart disease were not allowed to go to the dentist without the cover of an antibiotic. The concern was a condition called bacterial endocarditis (inflammation of the heart lining membrane). It led to brain abscesses and grim death.

Before antibiotics? The patient often just went and died; but of course the dentist never got blamed.

This risk factor is still true today. We still recommend antibiotic cover for patients with artificial heart valves, a previous history of endocarditis, certain congenital heart defects such as shunts, repaired congenital heart disease with prosthetic material or device and transplant cases. This is an authentic holistic physician talking: these people have to have antibiotics, for their very lives.

But I would amend it for my readers as follows: even really healthy people need to be aware of the risk to their arteries when undertaking dental care. If you are having any dental work done and you have infection problems in your teeth or gums, it's one of the few times when I would suggest you consider antibiotics for a couple of days. Don't fall for the idea of just one single huge dose. That's what I sometimes do and it's rather naughty. That's how we get resistant bacteria.

Now a very recent study (this month!) showed a correlation between poor teeth and cognitive decline in later years. Yet another reason to focus on oral health. The researchers were unable to conclude whether poor teeth or dentures led to a bad eating and thus poor nutrition, or whether poor dental hygiene and mental decline shared a common causative factor.

J Am Geriatr Soc. 2007 Sep;55(9):1410-4.

Heavy Metal Poisoning

Many people have become aware of the mercury toxicity problem. But it would be a mistake to think that metal poisoning is unique to this particular toxin. Consider: silver colloid is an antiseptic and has been used since ancient times to inhibit bacteria in drinking water. If it poisons germs, it will poison you. I have written elsewhere that iron forms the most destructive free-radical of all ("hot iron"), very damaging to life.

> **Metals can damage DNA, that means an increased risk of cancer!**

The fact is that all metals are toxic and our bodies require special transport and handling mechanisms to keep them from harming us. This applies just as much as essential minerals, like iron, zinc and chromium, as it does to non-essential metals and metalloids, like cadmium and arsenical compounds.

Heavy Metals and Cancer

A number of metals, and their compounds are known to be carcinogenic. These are:

- Arsenic
- Beryllium
- Cadmium
- Nickel
- Hexavalent chromium

The usual target is the lung, however cancer of the skin, and other cancers can be directly linked to heavy metals.

There are other metals which cause damage. Toxic metals can cause serious health problems by interruption normal biological function. While some can be found in the body in high concentration, many of these heavy metals - aluminum, beryllium, cadmium, lead and mercury, have no biological function. Arsenic, copper, iron and nickel are metals that are safe at low concentrations, but are toxic at high levels.

Heavy metals disrupt metabolic function in two basic ways. They accumulate and disrupt function in vital organs and glands; and they displace vital nutritional minerals from where they should be in the body to provide biological function. They impact at a foundational level, so they can be factors in any health problem.

Avoiding Heavy Metal Exposure is Impossible
Such preventative measures are futile. The reality is that it is impossible in our modern work to avoid exposure to heavy metals. So how do we get rid of heavy metal then? Chelation, which eliminates heavy metal poisons.

Sources of Heavy Metal
While this list provides many sources of the described metal, it's important to realize we could not include every possible source so be aware around you and when purchasing products. The side effects are far too many to list here as well. If you think you have heavy metal toxicity be sure to do your research.

ALUMINUM - aluminum foil, antacids, aspirin, beer, bleached flour, cans, ceramics, cheese, cigarette filters, color additives, construction materials, cookware, cosmetics, dental amalgams, deodorants, drinking water, pesticides, pollution, toothpaste.

Effects - ALS, Alzheimer's, anemia, appetite loss, behavioral problems, cavities, colitis, constipation, dementia, dry skin, energy loss, flatulence, headaches, heartburn, hyperactivity, kidney dysfunction, lowered immune function, learning disabilities, liver dysfunction, memory loss, numbness, osteoporosis, Parkinson's disease, peptic ulcer, stomach pain, weak and aching muscles.

ARSENIC - burning arsenate treated building materials, coal combustion, insect sprays, pesticides, seafood from coastal waters.

Effects - abdominal pain, anorexia, brittle nails, diarrhea, nausea, vomiting, chronic anemia, burning in mouth, esophagus, convulsions, dermatitis, drowsiness, hair loss, headaches, increased risk of liver/lung/skin cancers, low grade fever, muscle aches, nervousness, sweet metallic taste, throat constriction.

BERYLLIUM - coal burning, manufacturing, household products, industrial dust.

Effects - disturbance of calcium/vitamin D metabolism, magnesium depletion, lung infection, rickets, vital organ dysfunction.

CADMIUM - airborne industrial contaminants, batteries, candy, ceramics, cigarette smoke, colas, dental alloys, drinking water, electroplating, fertilizers, food from contaminated soil, processed foods, evaporated milk, motor oil, oysters, paint, pesticides, galvanized pipes, carpet backing, tobacco, vapor lamps, welding metal.

Effects - alcoholism, alopecia, anemia, arthritis, bone pain, cancer, cardiovascular disease, cavities, cirrhosis, diabetes, enlarged heart, flu-like symptoms, high cholesterol, hypertension, hypoglycemia, learning disorders, lung disease, migraines, schizophrenia, stroke.

COPPER - birth control pills, cookware, copper IUDs, copper pipes, dental alloys, fungicides, ice makers, industrial emissions, swimming pools, avocado, beer, chocolate, corn oil, crabs, lamb, margarine, milk, and many other foods.

Effects - acne, allergies, anemia, arthritis, autism, cancer, cystic fibrosis, depression, diabetes, fatigue, heart attack, high blood pressure, high cholesterol, Hodgkin's disease, hypertension, kidney disorders, mental illness, migraines, MS, nervousness, sexual dysfunction, stroke, toxemia of pregnancy, UTI, yeast infections.

IRON - drinking water, iron cookware, pipes, welding, many different foods:

Effects - anger, birth defects, bleeding gums, cancer, constipation, diabetes, dizziness, fatigue, headache, heart damage, insomnia, mental problems, metallic taste in mouth, nausea, pancreas damage, Parkinson's disease, schizophrenia, scurvy, shortness of breath, stubbornness.

LEAD - ash, auto exhaust, battery manufacturing, canned fruit and juice, car batteries, cigarette smoke, colored inks, cosmetics, utensils, household dust, glass production, hair dyes, lead pipes, milk, newsprint, pesticides, refineries, toothpaste, drinking water.

Effects - abdominal pain, anemia, anorexia, anxiety, arthritis, ADD, blindness, cardiovascular disease, concentration loss, constipation, convulsions, deafness, depression, epilepsy, immune suppression, decreased IQ, mood swings, muscle aches, muscle weakness, Parkinson's disease, psychosis, restlessness, retardation, schizophrenia, stillbirths, SID's, tingling, tooth decay, vertigo.

MERCURY - adhesives, air conditioner filters, algaecides, antiseptics, battery manufacturing, body powders, broken thermometers, cereals, dental amalgams, diuretics, fabric softeners, floor waxes, manufacture of paper and chlorine, medications, paints, pesticides, Preparation H, soft contact lens solution, tattooing.

Effects - adrenal dysfunction, allergy, birth defects, brain damage, cataracts, cerebral palsy, poor, deafness, depression, dermatitis, dizziness, drowsiness, fatigue, gum bleeding, hyperactivity, hypothyroidism, memory loss, mental retardation, migraines, numbness, pain in limbs, rashes, suicidal tendencies, tingling, weakness.

NICKEL - butter, fertilizers, food processing, fuel oil combustion, hydrogenated fats and oils, imitation whipped cream, industrial waste, kelp, margarine, nuclear device testing, oysters, stainless steel cookware, tea, tobacco smoke, unrefined grains and cereals, vegetable shortening.

Effects - anorexia, kidney dysfunction, apathy, disruption of hormone and lipid metabolism, fever, hemorrhages, headache, heart attack, intestinal cancer, low blood pressure, muscle tremors, nausea, oral cancer, skin problems, vomiting.

Persistence in the environment
One of the problems with metals is their environmental persistence. Once mined and brought into the ecology, they last almost indefinitely.

Also, we face the usually-ignored problem of potentiation, which means two relatively small doses of two different substances may have a dramatically enhanced effect when present together. For instance it is not widely known that the presence of lead (which is everywhere) makes mercury 100 times more toxic.

We call these metal-metal interactions and they might be quite critical in the formation of cancers. Animal studies also indicate, for example, that calcium enhances lead toxicity in rats and cadmium increases the likelihood of cadmium-induced prostatic cancer.

Given these insights, the complacency of traditional dentists over the cocktail of metalloids they put in our mouths as "amalgam" is little short of scientific folly. In the US they call them silver fillings, in an effort to imply purity and divert from the fact they are an amalgam of several different metals, of which silver is only a small proportion of the whole.

Protection From Other Metals
But it also works the other way. The presence of a second metal may actually protect against toxicity. Thus, for instance, magnesium was shown in animal studies to prevent cadmium-induced testicular tumors and zinc blocks lung cancer caused by continued inhalation of cadmium. Both magnesium and manganese were effective at preventing tumors which otherwise formed at the site of nickel injections in rats.

In fact magnesium has been shown to have a wide variety of beneficial effects against metal carcinogenesis risk factors. Yet another reason why magnesium is one of the most vital and health-giving nutrients we have. Avoid deficiency at all costs.

We have known for decades that selenium is vitally protective against mercury and also has a powerful anti-cancer benefit. When the daily intake is 100 microgrammes or more (200 mcg is better), the risk of cancer from all sources drops dramatically.

What Can You Do?
Apart from living in isolation on an organic farm, not much. And that's only relative. Don't be fooled that you would be safe in this environment; metals are in the air, as experience with strontium 90 and other radio-active atoms shows. Attempts to remove lead from our motor combustion engines is a good start. Better copper-based plumbing is also a right move.

But there is much pollution in the food chain. Lead dust is everywhere by the highways and in the dirt, left there from over a quarter of a century ago, when it was spewed by motor exhausts. Having an intelligent strategy to get rid of heavy metal poisons is critical to survival in the coming century and much wiser than wishing it wasn't there or wanting to run away to some transient utopia.

Do all you can to reduce the load by all means.

But rely more on competitive inhibition: that means the presence of "good" metals to squeeze out the bad ones. Remember all metals are toxic. But in reasonable physiological doses zinc, magnesium and selenium are important protectives. Fill up the seats with good guys and the bad guys can't enjoy the show.

You should be taking 200 mcg daily of selenium, 20-50 milligrams of zinc (citrate form is shown to be best absorbed) and 350 milligrams of magnesium, as the orotate, gluconate or amino-chelate. Watch out for diarrhea from magnesium salts, otherwise you might actually suffer a loss of mineral intake.

These will tend to squeeze the bad guys.

Chelation
DMPS, DMSA, KELMER and EDTA

Where the situation is serious, for example, lead or copper overload, I give IV ethyldiethylamine tetracetic acid (EDTA), in a series of infusions taking 3 hours or so each. The many benefits of this therapy can be read earlier in this book.

Unfortunately, this therapy is inadequate for mercury toxicity. There are three effective strategies for mercury, each with pros and cons:

6- 10 IV infusions of DMPS, 3 mgms per kg of body weight. These need skilled experience but done properly and at the correct dose I find have virtually no side-effects. The theoretical risk here is that DMPS crosses the blood-brain barrier and may carry mercury into neurological tissues, where it is most unwelcome. Side effects can be unpleasant and this seems the least advisable method.

Oral DMSA, 30 mgms per kg body weight. Duration depends on response but in the region of 6-10 weeks. Side effects can be unpleasant but can be ameliorated by reducing the dose. Generally children tolerate DMSA much better than adults.

Oral chelation with magnesium succinate (*marketed as Kelmer), 60 mg per kg body weight. I am satisfied that this produces the same degree of mercury elimination as DMSA but without the unwanted side effects. It just takes longer, is all!

There is controversy over whether EDTA will remove mercury. For all sorts of scientific reasons, to do with valence and electrical charge, it shouldn't work well. But Dr Gary Gordon claims is does: by actual urine and tissue testing, that it can be seen being excreted after his oral chelation regime (which admittedly includes a lot more than mere EDTA).

Self-administered therapy is not recommended. But chlorella is a great heavy metal attractor, is safe and plentiful. Lesser players are garlic and cilantro.

Finally, remember that once the source of contamination is removed, if you support your body with good detox and nutritional requirements, the heavy metals will gradually disappear from the tissues by slow attrition, a process termed leaching or, more exactly, depuration.

Intestinal Metal Detox (IMD)

This is a revolutionary product group developed by young boffin Christopher Shade. It's called "intestinal" metal detox because, factually, that's where most toxic metal excretion takes place.

The problem is these toxic metals inflame the gut lining, which causes it to leak, and so we re-absorb of lot of the excreted toxins. This is hardly helpful.

One of the critical services provided by Shade's labs (Quicksilver Scientific) is mercury speciation; that means identifying the relative load of different "species" of mercury:

norganic mercury (Hg^{II})
methylmercury (MeHg)
total mercury (Hg^{II} + MeHg)
ethylmercury (expanded speciation analysis only)
other forms (dimethylmercury, propylmercury, etc.)

Each of these forms behaves differently and total mercury load may give no real guidance to the type of mercury overload, where it is found in the body and how to get rid of it.

Quicksilver Scientific's testing takes care of this danger and uncertainty, which I why I approve of them.

To date, Quicksilver Scientific is the only commercial analysis company whose laboratory has the capability to directly analyze ethylmercury, methylmercury, and inorganic mercury in one simultaneous procedure at environmentally and biologically relevant amounts.

Find out more at: http://www.quicksilverscientific.com

Laughter And Play
People don't laugh enough. A good belly laugh every day can save your life.

In 1979 Norman Cousins surprised us all with his revelation that he had all but recovered from a crippling and life-threatening collagen disease, using laughter. He followed a regimen of high doses of Vitamin C and of positive emotions, including daily doses of belly laughs, which he brought on using comedy movies.

Cousins chronicled his recovery in the best-selling Anatomy of an Illness. In the book, generalizing from his own experience and research, he affirmed that "the life force may be the least understood force on earth" and that "human beings are not locked into fixed limitations. The quest for perfectibility is not a presumption or a blasphemy but the highest manifestation of a great design."

Did you know that kids laugh about 400 time's day, while adults only laugh a measly 25 times? There is a message here: if you want boundless energy like kids have, no matter your age, laugh and play like kids do. Get down and dirty! Muss your hair, scuff your knees; what does it matter?

You Can Do More:

1. Tell jokes. Make people laugh. You'll laugh yourself as a result.

2. Smile. Tests carried out by Robert Holden and BBC2 showed that even just smiling at yourself in the mirror is uplifting.

> **A good belly laugh every day can save your life.**

3. Play with your kids. Well, if you're past that, play with the grandkids! Or play with a pet. Goldfish aren't much fun but cats and dogs can be.

4. Dance. Well, I've already covered that above. Add some hop, skip and jumps once a day! Who cares if people think you are nuts? How crazy do you have to be to enjoy life and want to live longer, huh?

5. Go back to a favorite hobby; something you used to really love doing. Make time for it a few hours a week, come what may. Instead of thinking of wasting time, thinking of it as harvesting back years that you would have lost, due to early death.

Notice I'm talking real play, not sport. The difference is that in sport you are committed to the outcome (winning). With play, you don't need to care about winning. Having a good time is winning.

15 | Love And Sex

There is no question that life energy and sexual vibrancy are inter-related (causally). More and more science is being found to educate us that sex can mitigate the effects of stress, lead to a happier life, more balanced emotions and continued physical vigor.

Even if you are not in an active relationship, masturbation is considered healthy and useful (and certainly not shameful), to bring you a quota of the magical and inspiring sensation we call an orgasm. Both men and women should masturbate if they can't have an orgasm any other way.

Sorry if this shocks you, but God gave you the faculty of self-effected orgasm, not me! I'm only reporting the facts. Masturbation (coyly called "self-cultivation" on an Oprah Winfrey show) is the most common form of sexuality, despite people's inhibitions talking about it and doing it.

Men, you will learn, have less prostatic disease if they masturbate regularly. Women are more likely to have fulfilling sex lives, better health, better marriages, and an overall increase in self-confidence. Masturbation for both sexes is associated with improved cardiovascular health and lower risk of type-2 diabetes.

Anybody have a problem with that? I don't. Science is telling us that the party poopers who tell you it's wicked are spouting bad science, even if they try to cover their guilt and folly with religious authority. Nature loves you!

Vitamin L

Have you heard of vitamin L? It's love! It could be laughter or light. One way or another, light brings us life. The sun's energy is converted to sugars by green plants; these are eaten by animals, which obtain energy. That includes humans, of course.

But love is the missing ingredient in many lives and we have a poor and undernourished state of health without it. Love enriches; love makes us more ourselves. Love brings warmth and purpose and creative energy. It diminishes pain and makes suffering more bearable. It is the single greatest human "feel good" factor on earth. We mean here interpersonal love, affinity and friendship, not romantic sexual love. That may certainly be included but children, old folk, anyone living singly can share in love.

Man is basically a friendly animal. Our biological order, the apes, are all group-oriented species. We belong with them and share many characteristics, including this one.

Now scientists have managed to prove what we all knew - the power of love. Individuals shown classic mushy love movies had significantly increased levels of protective antibodies. One may infer that they would live longer in this state, less likely to fall foul of disease.

Another study showed that people in love have less poisonous lactic acid and higher levels of feel-good endorphins in their blood. But probably the best proof came from a famous study of 10,000 male heart patients in Israel in 1976. Researchers found that patients were far less likely to have dangerous heart symptoms if they could answer "Yes!" to the simple question: does your wife show you she loves you?

That love is an important factor in longevity is shown by the studies of Professor Pitzkhelauri of the Caucasus region and reported by Alexander Leaf MD in National Geographic January 1973. The Georgians and Azerbaijanis of this region are noted for their extreme longevity and rival, or even surpass, the famous Hunzas of northern Pakistan.

Ages of 100-120 were far from rare; indeed the average man expected to live to 100 years and many did better than this. The Soviet research, examining figures of 15,000 persons over 80, showed that with rare exceptions, only married couples attained extreme ages. Many couples have been married 70, 80 or even 100 years. Marriage and a regular prolonged sex life are very important to longevity, Professor Pitzkhelauri concluded.

It can also protect from degenerative change. Destructive cortisol levels (**page 26**) were higher in monkeys kept deprived of parental contact. In human terms, there is an 8% increase in the chances of Alzheimer's disease (AD) for every additional child in a family.

A 1999 study published in the medical journal Neurology showed that stable married individuals were far less likely to develop Alzheimer's than those who were not. It even showed that those who were divorced or widowed were protected to some degree, proving the old adage that it is better to have loved and lost than never to have loved at all.

The moral for those who want to live longer and avoid the degenerative brain changes of aging is **get plenty of love**. Now we all know the irony that as time goes by, the magic of romantic love tends to fade. But core love never goes away, indeed it seems to grow as the years pass. What seems to be important is the expression of love in our lives. You may have lived with the same person for many years and lost the habit of saying "I love you". The idea of starting to use these words once more may seem scary.

But if you can revive the habit, you'll live longer. That's a pretty positive transaction; a far better deal than any you could get on the stock exchange!

What Can You Do?

There is an old line: *fake it till you make it*. Even if you don't feel much love, create it anyway and real love will start to emerge. How can you do that?

- You can sing happy songs and love songs, songs of the heart
- You can think about things you really love (not necessarily people)
- Start to show more compassion and care for others and it will come back to you
- If you are not already in the habit, use the word LOVE as often as you can. To say it out loud gives it a strange power that exceeds merely thinking about it.

Finally, if your key life relationship has gone sour, what can you do? Well, you loved the person once. You had better try again. Just to hold in your mind endless bitterness and criticism of your life partner will shorten your life as sure as drink and smoking. Bitterness kills. Try at least to acknowledge more positive things about the significant other. To hold them in contempt diminishes you and may cause you to feel stupid or paltry.

Remember, you get back what you give out.
If the relationship has become so sick as to be destructive, you must correct it or get out. It is always harder if only one of the two is honest and striving to make things work better. Just don't ignore it any longer. Hurt, suffering and strife (all manifestations of stress) will raise your cortisol levels and shorten your life.

If things are so bad you cannot imagine being able to get back to a good place, try Co-Dependents Anonymous (CoDA). You can make contact with a branch via the Internet through www.codependents.org.

HOT TIP

We don't owe love and nobody owes us. But there are those who we know in our hearts deserve our love and, so often, we haven't the courage or initiative to tell them so. Don't wait for the deathbed scene! So many loving individuals bring this message to a dying partner, parent, friend or family member. If you know you need to say it, SAY IT NOW! Get it over with. Then you can enjoy the remaining times of goodness and good cheer.

Just do it!
Make sure you visit to the Web site of the Institute of Heart Math in Boulder Creek, California. It is a non-profit research organization that is filled with many "heart scientists," dedicated to researching the power of the heart to transform lives for the better. Their larger mission is to help change the world and make it a safer gentler place for all.

That Loving Touch
Now there is science to prove what we all knew – that a loving touch feels good but also calms and allays our fears and pain. The corroborative evidence comes from an interesting study, using brain scans to monitor emotional responses, headed by Dr. James Coan, a psychologist in the departments of psychology and neuroscience at the University of Virginia.

The basic set up was that women were put into an MRI scanner and told to expect mild electrical shocks applied to their ankles. Enough to make anyone tense and anxious (this study did not address the fact that MRI scanners, quite independently of the electrical shocks, induce deep fear and nausea in many people).

But, the scientists found, if the husband is brought into the picture and allowed to hold his wife's hand, she calms down and relaxes. The pain even goes away. And it was all monitored on the scanner. Proof! Even a stranger's hand worked some magic apparently but there was no question: that love was the powerful factor and hubby's hand was better than any other. The stronger the bond between the couple, as assessed by a pre-test questionnaire, the more pronounced the calming and soothing effect of the loved one's touch.

Brain images showed peaks of activation in regions involved in anticipating pain, heightening physical arousal and regulating negative emotions, among other systems. But when holding hands, the signals markedly declined in intensity. The volunteers also said that they felt less distress.

"The effect of this simple gesture of social support is that the brain and body don't have to work as hard, they're less stressed in response to a threat," said Dr. James A. Coan, the study's lead author. His co-authors were Dr. Hillary Schaefer and Dr. Richard J. Davidson of the University of Wisconsin.

> **A loving touch feels good but also calms and allays our fears and pain.**

The findings go some way to explain the well-documented fact that married men and women are healthier on average than their peers. Husbands and wives who are close tend to limit each other's excesses like drinking and smoking but that's not enough to account for their better health compared with singles, researchers say.

There is some other fact at work and it is clearly a measurable reality. Loving healthy couples keep each other calmer and out of harm's way. Lowering stress is one of the most important ways to live longer and avoid sickness.

From which we may conclude that it is healthy and prophylactic (preventative) to hug and kiss, to touch amorously, and to re-affirm verbally and visually that you love one another.

If yours is not the kind of relationship which elicits this sort of behavior then beware: you will not reap the benefits but, more to the point, the relationship may be a source of stress, not a preventative.

Women Are The Health Sentries
Men, we all know, are pathetic when it comes to taking care of themselves. Their usual response to symptoms and danger signs is complete denial. Women pay careful attention to their husbands' well-being, pick up signals and symptoms, and get their men to the doctor. Put simply, most men depend exclusively on their wives to monitor, medicate, nurse and nudge them—in the here-and-now and through their waning years.

But now there is this extra factor. That wifely nurturing after a fallout with a neighbor or a thrashing in the boardroom could work as well as a tranquilizer or a beta-blocker.

Having a partner helps men with cancer—specifically, cancer of the prostate or bladder—survive longer and with a better quality of life, according to studies at the Jonsson Comprehensive Cancer Center at UCLA.

The same is true for men hospitalized with heart disease: In a study at the University of California at San Diego, coronary-bypass patients whose wives visited them early and often in the intensive-care unit required less pain medication and recovered more quickly than men without a spouse. Conversely, the patients whose wives did not provide much emotional support fared worse.

Love is the Key

Evidence is mounting dramatically that the quality of a marriage is strongly related to the health of both partners. In fact, a man who has a secure marriage and who continues to be sexually active lives longer, succumbs to illness less often and heals from wounds and surgery faster. Why? Because he is insulated from stress by love.

The wiring circuits for emotion in the brain, the limbic system, is situated directly next to—and are deeply connected to—the hypothalamic system that control heart rate, blood pressure and how much adrenaline one secretes. "You can see the two circuits talking to each other on imaging machines," says Dr. Harry Lodge, an internist in New York City and co-author of Younger Next Year. "A bad emotional state makes needles jump. A really good marriage is harder to measure—it's an absence of those jumps."

Unfortunately, there is an inevitable downside to all this lovie-dovie: if the couple is continuously in strife, quarrelling with each other and holding onto cold hostile attitudes instead of love that hurts health and can slow the process of healing. In an experiment conducted by Drs. Janice Kiecolt-Glaser and Ronald Glaser at Ohio State University, long-married couples were given minor blister wounds, and then asked to discuss a disagreement. Compared to the harmonious couples, the hostile couples took up to two days longer to heal.

Likewise, cardiologists report that if there is an undercurrent of hostility or resentment in a marriage or a suspicion of extramarital affairs, the whole cardiac recovery process slows down.

Only secure and happy marriages reap the rewards of better health and longevity. Take heed!

Sex Matters

We would all like to go on finding or I should say rediscovering love in our partner and ourselves. Sexual vitality is important and its health benefits cannot be overestimated. And I don't mean the love of a rich old boy for a young flirt or a woman who is loaded after her husband's death suddenly finding herself surrounded by admirers. You know the sort of thing...

What I am talking about is the real honest deep-down passion for the companion who has shared your life and whom you want to continue to admire and cherish. Someone you want to hang onto and you wish they were happy and well, as you would wish it just for yourself. Or if he or she is no longer with you in life, that you can re-find yourself and live with new devotion and love that he or she would have wanted to you enjoy.

I'm not talking here about "twilight" years, so much as the dawn of a new day!

When all is said and done, a solid marriage with regular and enthusiastic sex can be the best preventive medicine of all. In a woman, repeated affectionate hugs release the "bonding hormone" oxytocin and reduce blood pressure, which helps to protect her heart. In men, the levels of oxytocin can and do surge up to five times above normal, but only immediately before he reaches orgasm – well, that's guys for you. We need that special moment, ladies - it keeps us alive!

In a study at Queen's University in Belfast, the mortality of about 1,000 middle-aged men of comparable health was tracked over the course of a decade. The men who had sex three or more times a week had a 50% reduced risk of heart attack or stroke. And those who reported the most frequent orgasms had a death rate one-half that of the less sexually active men.

Can you imagine the response of doctors to a drug that cut the death rate in half? They'd go wild with excitement. Yet here is a simple prescription (love) that would do just that and it never gets mentioned. Has your doctor ever even asked you if you were in love, happy and having fulfilling sex?

No, I thought not.

Sex Releases Stress
(But we all knew that, didn't we?)

Got some public speaking to do? Driving test? Exams? Here is a surprise tip to reduce the feelings of stress: have sex beforehand. But make sure it's penetrative sex - the magic vanishes if you pursue other forms of sexual gratification (apparently).

Stuart Brody, a psychologist at the University of Paisley (outside Glasgow), UK, compared the impact of different sexual activities on blood pressure when a person later experiences acute stress. For a fortnight, 24 women and 22 men kept diaries of how often they engaged in penile-vaginal intercourse (PVI), masturbation or partnered sexual activity excluding intercourse. After, the volunteers underwent a stress test involving public speaking and mental arithmetic out loud.

Volunteers who'd had PVI but none of the other kinds of sex were least stressed, and their blood pressure returned to normal faster than those who'd only masturbated or had non-coital sex. Those who abstained had the highest blood-pressure response to stress (Biological Psychology, Vol. 71, p 214).

Brody also made psychological measurements of neuroticism and anxiety in the volunteers, as well as work stress and partnership satisfaction. Even taking these factors into account, differences in sexual behavior provided the best explanation for the range of stress responses. "The effects are not attributable simply to the short-term relief afforded by orgasm, but rather, endure for at least a week," says Brody. He speculates that release of the "pair-bonding" hormone oxytocin between partners might account for the calming effect.

Of course there may be another reason Brody is missing. Penetrative sex may only be a regular option among couples who are already stable, centered and affectionate. This is still the same basic message, which is that the biology of love shows sex to be natural, healthy and healing. There are many studies which have shown that couples in love have sustained positive health benefits on each other.

This may be one of the reasons solid couples live longer and are healthier maybe.

Remember also the controversial first issue (now archived in the members' area) in which I described the scientific health benefits of masturbation. Maybe the free love, abundant sex era of the 60s was such a good health foundation that it is why the baby boomers (who were doin' it then!) are now living so long!

The Midlife Crisis

The menopause is a well-known event for women, even celebrated, though this has been late in coming to the understanding of men -- and male doctors in particular. What is much less known is that men have to endure a similar biological and emotional experience. It is obscured by the usual male inability to come to terms with personal issues and the fact that it is perceived as less than masculine to even admit to such feelings.

Matters are made more complicated by the fact that there are really two phenomena rolled into one and these easily become confused. It is vital that women appreciate what is happening to their loved one and that doctors get to grips with this important aspect of growing older.

Although men like to believe they are tough and immune from care, the truth is they are often desperately insecure and failing to understand what is happening to one's self can be a major cause of anxiety and suffering.

There is a male hormonal shut-down, akin to the menopause, which is therefore named the "andropause". But this is quite distinct from the mid-life crisis, as we shall see in detail. The trouble is that both happen at a similar time, though the crucial difference is that the mid-life crisis tends to occur somewhat earlier. How can we tell these two apart?

Let us consider first the true andropause.

Characteristics Of The Andropause

It starts, usually, in the fifth decade. It is unrelated to life events (though it may happen at the same time as an unrelated disaster). There are true biological changes, which can be measured in the laboratory. Testosterone levels fall. The resulting symptoms are not unlike those experienced by a woman at the menopause:

- fatigue

- depression
- aches and pains
- sweating and flushes
- reduced libido

To which may be added: loss of erectile function. The latter is particularly disturbing to a man and difficulty in talking about this problem is one of the reasons why the male menopause has been little attended to.

The True Mid-Life Crisis

This often falls earlier than the andropause, maybe in the fourth decade. Typically, it occurs in response to some outside challenge in a man's life: a breakdown of the marriage, career failure, bankruptcy, death of a peer or loved parent, redundancy and so on. Essentially, it is an emotional crisis and not a hormonal one.

Deep introspection often results in the feeling that life is passing by and precious years have been wasted with so little achieved. Dreams that were once so important seem to have faded or gone forever beyond reach. It can be a time of great anguish, despair, inadequacy and feelings of guilt or futility.

Whereas anyone, sooner or later, will experience a shutdown of hormones, the man who suffers the mid-life crisis is typically one who has been challenged and cannot come to terms with his life. There has been a shock, which brings him face to face with self and he doesn't like what he sees.

In trying to rationalize the unhappy feelings he may begin to see his life partner in negative terms or blame his bosses and work dissatisfaction. Therefore he seeks change: a new partner (times of infidelity and experiment), a new career, new home territory and so on.

Unfortunately, alcohol and drugs are often seen as the answer. They shut out the pain temporarily but of course solve nothing. This may be the start of a slippery slope to abuse, addiction and early demise.

Far from the libido shut down characteristic of the andropause, a man in a mid-life crisis wants to boast of sexual prowess and seeks new thrills and adventure. This is the man likely to start buying younger generation fashion clothes and run off with a tart or have an affair with his secretary in her twenties. But it is a kind of denial, an admission that things are not as they were, underscored by a great desire to prove everything is OK, "No problem!"

The andropause man lacks any energy or drive and cannot be bothered with sex or adventure. For him, it already is too late (he thinks).

What Lies Beyond

One can gain a deeper insight by looking far beyond the moment of crisis. The mid-life crisis is a kind of rite of passage. It comes to an end eventually and good may come of it. A marriage may not always be wrecked but may be strengthened and renewed by surviving the threat. A great deal depends on the response of the life partner in this time of upheaval and change.

A man may be renewed through suffering, discover a vision for the future and come home once again to feelings of family and love. He can learn something of great value, about himself, about others, about the deeper nature of life. If the trigger was a financial collapse, he may recover the determination to work hard and rebuild his empire. In this way, some men will go forward and meet the challenge.

Sadly, many do not do so but give in to what they see as an overwhelming tide of misfortune. Alcohol or drug addiction takes a lasting grip. These individuals rapidly advance into the inertia of age and decrepitude. For them, the mid-life crisis was a disaster from which they do not recover.

Women

And yes, the mid-life crisis can occur for women. Almost all of what is said here applies equally. Even the search for new loves, thrills and adventure can lead to women also becoming unfaithful or seeking divorce. Obviously it needs to be distinguished from the onset of the menopause.

The trouble is women often give up their lives to children and then, when the children leave, they don't know what to do. They have given themselves to the children, at the expense often of a loving relationship with the husband. By then it is TOO LATE to restart things with the husband. Sad story of most marriages!

What You Can Do

The most important first step is to have blood tests to check up on the man's hormones, as described in the chapter HORMONES FOR MEN and PROSTATE. If this reveals there is a problem, testosterone supplements are needed and will work a satisfying and sometimes dramatic change. The fatigue and depression will lift, life becomes worthwhile, energy levels and zest return to former levels, potency problems recede.

What is more, testosterone improves circulation, protects against heart disease, aids weight loss, improves skin condition, increases muscle strength and works in a host of healthy ways to rejuvenate the man. It is a tragedy that early experiments (with artificial methyl testosterone) bungled by the greed of drug companies have led to testosterone supplements having bad press.

Testosterone supplementation does need some care and is discussed elsewhere. Generally, though, one can say that the dangers of NOT supplementing testosterone well into old age are far greater than any theoretical risks to prescribing it. Be clear about it: **testosterone saves lives and saves hearts and minds!** (see page 113)

On the other hand, what if the tests show that testosterone deficiency is not significant? Clearly, supplements will not help. This is an emotional or life-events crisis and needs handling as such, at whatever age it befalls.

The first sensible step towards surviving the mid-life crisis is having the problem identified and understood, as above. Kindness, tact and sympathy are required, despite outrageous and often destructive behavior by the affected individual, because it is still a medical condition.

Any crisis is a time of great stress and stress, we know, is a killer. It shortens lives. If the individual is already abusing drugs and drink as a solution, then the danger to health and longevity is even greater. Bitter acrimony and rejection from relatives, even though badly affected in turn, are counter-productive, and simply make everyone suffer more. At all costs, keep the communication flowing; it's the only hope for a sane future and rebuilding friendships.

The man concerned has to be brought to confronting his situation. The pretense that there is nothing wrong and everyone else is to blame does not help. Dr Malcolm Carruthers, a male hormone and lifestyle specialist and author of *The Testosterone Revolution* makes the point that the kind of man likely to suffer a mid-life crisis is one with an unhappy childhood, maybe abusive or with cold and unloving parents. Such early formative experiences often engender a feeling of unworthiness which emerges later in life, at a time of crisis. This is fruitful ground for counseling or other therapy.

Even without a therapist, a man can sit down with pen and paper and start to write down *what matters*. Nothing changes the meaning of life more than working out what one's values truly are. Often we aspire to false goals, imposed by others, which have little meaning to ourselves.

Society at large, and the media in particular, often impose ridiculous standards of goodness and value. There is a cult of greed, materialism and celebrity worship in vogue which is very dangerous and tends to create envy, desire, inadequacy and misery in those who do not have all the trappings of a luxurious film-star lifestyle.

The irony is, you only have to look at the stories in that same press to realize that the people we are supposed to envy have disastrous, miserable and often very short sick lives.

Pueraria mirifica, a herbal remedy from Thailand, Herbal Remedy From Thailand

Pueraria mirifica (also known as Kwao Krua or Butea Superba; see page 118) is a plant found only in Thailand and parts of Burma; 99% is grown in Thailand. Menopausal women, have been using Pueraria Mirifica for 700 years.

The region where this plant is grown is remarkable for its low rate of breast cancer and impressive longevity, which alerted scientists to something good going on. The lucky women get to use this local plant and the benefits are enormous and the science is building all the time.

Men should use it too, especially as they age, since men are increasingly exposed to old-age estrogens ("male estrogen").

The active ingredients seem to be miroestrol and deoxymiroestrol. These have been shown to be 3,000 more potent as estrogens than soy isoflavones and, according to Dr. Garry Gordon MD, Pueraria mirifica "Makes Black Cohosh and Red Clover look like placebos."

Mirifica means "miracle" and it seems as if we have a miracle herb on our hands.

There is no increase in estrogen levels ever found, yet it reverses atrophic vaginitis and in fact, Dr. Christiane Northrup has reported that vaginal tissues become years younger and painful intercourse disappears. It is also available for topical use to apply to the labia for quicker results, as Tigress PM.

The Problem

What Problem? Well, it is an estrogen mimic and ought to make estrogen dominance worse. But the fact it is doesn't. This blessed little herb is truly a gift to women tormented by their hormones (the majority). It works by attaching to estrogen receptors, so that real estrogen is rendered ineffective, but it does so without stimulating the receptors in a dangerous way.

This is sometimes called estrogen inhibition.

It actually works as well as the drug Tamoxifen, to reduce risk of breast cancer cells proliferating. There is much more to research on this incredible story, which it appears should be in the diet of every women from adolescence on, so that we bring breast cancer rates down to those in Northern Thailand, which is proven to be the lowest in the world.

Selective Estrogen Receptor Modulators (SERMs)

Pueraria in one of a group of emergent compounds, which includes the drug Tamoxifen, called selective estrogen receptor modulators or SERMs.

SERMs are called "selective" because they bind to particular estrogen receptors. SERMs do not prevent the production of estrogen, but they help to slow or stop the growth of estrogen-sensitive cancer cells by starving them of a full dose of natural estrogen.

There are other beneficial side effects, such as lowering cholesterol and protecting bone health for post-menopausal women, keeping the skeleton and joints strong and preventing breaks and fractures.

The latest remarkable discovery is that SERMs can protect your telomeres and that is a number one result for anti-aging (more of that in a moment).

Men Too!

Men can benefit too. We know that male estrogen increases through time, while testosterone falls, due to aging, body fat, hormonal replacement, pesticides, nutritional deficiencies, prescription medications and excessive alcohol intake. It's a condition called estrogen dominance.

In fact, studies have shown that the estrogen levels of the average 54-year-old man is higher than those of the average 59-year-old women! The end result is that these high levels of estrogen can cause reduced levels of testosterone, fatigue, loss of muscle tone, increased body fat, loss of libido and sexual function, an enlarged prostate and male titties [did you know that male breast reduction surgery is the fastest growing surgical procedures in the USA right now?]

So Pueraria has potential benefits for men too. It does not produce male breasts and may actually reduce this sign of aging plumpness.

But don't suppose PM will take the place of good diet, exercise, cutting down on alcohol and losing plenty of weight.

Reversing Aging

This is the bit we are interested in here.

Harvard scientists have taken prematurely aged mice and reversed the toll of time – increasing the size of their shrunken brains, restoring their diminished sense of smell, and turning their graying fur to a healthy sheen.

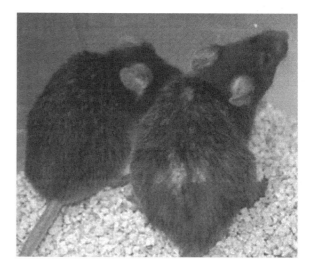

They did this by using the SERM properties.

The mice were at the very end of their lives and scientists expected no more than to slow or perhaps stabilize the aging process. Instead, they saw a dramatic reversal in the symptoms of aging.

The mice were specially developed to be telomere-deficient and aged fast. Just mid-way through the normal lifespan of a mouse, their organs had atrophied, their brains had shrunk, their coats turned gray and shabby and they had lost the ability to detect noxious odors.

But when scientists used a Tamoxifen-clone enzyme to switch the gene back on for a month, many hallmarks of aging seemed to reverse. The fertility of the mice increased, their sense of smell was restored, and their organs were rejuvenated. They literally went into aging reverse. (See photo. The mouse on the left once looked like the old crock on the right!)

Well, the complex enzyme used for this trial is not available commercially and I could not recommend Tamoxifen as a good idea, even if you could get your doctor to prescribe it.

But you can take Pueraria and expect at least some of this beneficial aging effect. In several senses, Pueraria mirifica is a "fountain of youth". Plus it's a lot cheaper than TA-65, at around $800 a month for four capsules a day.

Dosage and Sources

Menstruating Women
Daily doses of 100 mg to 600 mgs/day, following our current recommended schedule of the 8th day from the start of the monthly menstrual cycle to the 21st day.

Post-Menopausal Women
Daily dosing, with no cycle.

Men
Daily dosing, around 100 mg, with no cycle.

Sum Up Properties Of Pueraria Mirifica
1. slowing the aging process: anti-wrinkle agent; hair darkener, strengthener, and growth promoter
2. breast firming
3. counter-acting memory loss
4. alleviating cataract and other vision problems
5. increasing energy, vigor, flexibility
6. increasing blood circulation
7. increasing appetite
8. alleviating sleep disorders
9. preventing and aiding rehabilitation from strokes
10. alleviating the effects of menopause
11. restoring vaginal health and elasticity
12. countering osteoporosis
13. slowing and preventing prostate enlargement in men
14. preventing/mitigating dementia
15. Note the form known as Butea superba (in Thai, kwao kreu daeng) increases libido and sexual vitality for men.

Truly, a "miracle" herb and deserves its name.

16 | Engine Speed. The Thyroid Gland.

The big dividing line in healing philosophy between staid conventional colleagues and doctors like myself, is that we believe the patient more than they believe laboratory tests. If there is a conflict, we assume the patient is a more accurate monitor of disease than blood tests. I mean, how crazy is it to state to a patient (happens often) that, "We have done all the tests and there is nothing wrong," when the patient says she feels awful?

Take the treatment and investigation of thyroid disease as an example.

Doctors who don't think for themselves, but rely solely on the blood tests, will ignore striking symptoms such as fatigue, depression, sensitivity to cold, weight-gain, dry skin, hair loss in a middle-aged or older person, if the thyroid markers are "normal". Really dumb doctors might put it all down to "aging". But good holistic doctors will follow the symptoms and treat the clinical condition, which clearly exists.

The fact is that up to 20% of the population is probably suffering from some degree of hypothyroidism (low thyroid function), though in some territories it could be much higher. The opposite - hyperthyroidism, or overactivity of the gland - is actually relatively rare. The older you get, the more prone you are to the condition; it's part of natural aging. But it is still pathological and it should be treated!

Part of the problem is that the tests are pretty crude and disease has to become serious in degree before it shows up as altered blood levels. Also the usually quoted range is so wide it is relatively meaningless and you could be 50% down on "average" and still said to be within normal limits.

The real point is that a person can be functionally hypothyroid without any other abnormal markers than symptoms and signs of disease. It's a test of a doctor's skill to recognize and treat the disease they see, whether or not the laboratory is helpful in confirming the diagnosis.

It is vital that all doctors start to think more often of thyroid problems. Because it's not just a "quality of life" issue: your risk of heart disease is significantly increased and the confusion and lethargy which comes on may even be mistaken for senility and the patient put on a completely inappropriate program.

Immunity

What very few doctors seem to know is that the thyroid gland is wrapped up in the process of immunity. Several studies have shown that a patient with thyroid problems is more likely to develop cancer (cancer is best considered a disease of the immune system). This doesn't mean only thyroid cancer - any cancer could be involved!

I first came across the connection between thyroid and immunity in my work as an allergy guru. Time and again patients would present the symptoms of thyroid disease, along with their allergy problems. This was especially true of women and there is a very good reason. Women have a high incidence of a clinical condition called Hashimoto's disease (auto-immune thyroiditis), in which the body makes antibodies against the thyroid gland and hormones. It's one of those allergy-against-yourself diseases (rheumatoid arthritis is another).

It must be mentioned in passing that there is another kind of thyroiditis. This is not caused by antibodies but a virus, typically mumps or Coxsackie. Usually it resolves clinically but may be the source of chronic hypothyroidism.

Pioneer the late Dr Broda O. Barnes reckoned that hypothyroidism underpinned a huge range of diseases in the West, from heart disease, to allergies; cancer to apparent parasitism; loss of sexual function to visual acuity. Notice, by the way, how those are like a catalogue of aging problems!

But it's not just about pseudo-aging: for women, all kinds of menstrual difficulties—notably heavy flow—can be attributed to hypothyroidism, as can emotional and behavior problems in children. Indeed, there is a clear link between hypothyroidism and autism spectrum disorder.

Accelerating Problem

What's worrying is the theory that thyroid disorders are getting worse with every generation. One of the important reasons for such widespread hypothyroid problems in Western civilization is the fact that it is in large part due to the toxic overload that we all bear.

Nothing suffers quite so much as the thyroid gland from loading with pesticides, pollutants and toxic heavy metals. With each generation, the toxic overload accumulates steadily, much like chemicals accumulate moving up the food chain (remember, we are at the top of many food chains).

But the thyroid dysfunction multiplies too; each parent generation starting their kids off with an already compromised organ, who pass it on to their kids, even more disadvantaged still—and so it goes on.

If this is true, we would be facing thyroid misery of almost epidemic proportions. And you know what? That's exactly what we are seeing. But the medical profession is not getting it—because they rely entirely on stupid and unworkable test; nothing shows, so there is "no problem".

The Broda Barnes Temperature Test

Blood tests for thyroid hormones are totally unreliable; a patient may have normal thyroid hormone levels but, if the body is not responding to those hormones, a deficiency equivalent is the result.

A simple test for thyroid function which is very helpful is to take regular measurements of basal temperature - the so-called Broda Barnes test, named after the doctor who first wrote about it.

Basal temperature means while at absolute rest. In ordinary terms that means first thing on waking, after the body has been lying still overnight. Temperature drops to its lowest at this point. To measure your own basal temperature, use a clinical thermometer, keep it under your tongue, before getting out of bed or any activity whatsoever, for at least three minutes without opening your mouth. Record the results.

Generally, if it is running at 36.50 C (97.50 F) or less, that is presumptive evidence of low thyroid function. Allowance may need to be made for women who are ovulating, since the temperature naturally rises about 0.5 of a degree at this time. I will help the patient interpret what is found.

Other Tests

Bio-energetic testing, such as electro-acupuncture, may be yet another route by which poor thyroid function is called to the attention of the physician.

This also often shows us that other hormonal disturbance is present too, even if subtle and represented only at the energetic level. Furthermore we often learn that these hormone disruptions are the results of long standing energetic "shadows", some of which go back to childhood illnesses and vaccinations.

All very controversial.

But fortunately the new magic of electronic bio-energetic testing (see my latest book VIRTUAL MEDICINE from Thorsons) also often shows us effective herbal, homeopathic and other holistic remedies which will work in the presence of a hypothyroid problem.

Treatment

I my practice I use a several-fold approach. The simplest, if the signs are early enough and the patient is otherwise vigorous, is homeopathic thyroid stimulant. I use a product called Thyroidea compositum from Germany. It is one of the most powerful and useful non-drug substances I have in my repertoire. Such is its impact on immunity I find myself prescribing it often for my cancer patients seeking alternative remedies.

If a trial of this substance and related compounds appears ineffective, then supplementation with the hormone can be considered. Conventional colleagues would not normally approach things this way, feeling that if the blood levels are adequate then supplementation is pointless.

The stupidity of this attitude is that they then have nothing to offer the patient, beyond palliative treatment. Often this means prescribing anti-depressants for the lethargy and giving him or her a good ticking off about being overweight!

A better approach is to use what we call a "therapeutic trial". The patient then becomes his or her own test bed. If taking the hormone results in a rapid return to normal, with renewed zest and loss of weight encumbrance, is that not adequate intellectual evidence that the thyroid was indeed, in some way, under-performing?

Synthetic vs. Natural Replacement

The usual thyroid hormone (levothyroxine) is synthetically produced. There are sometimes considerations that make the natural product better. This means supplementing dried thyroid extract from animal sources (pig instead of beef, because of BSE). But if Hashimoto's disease is the problem, synthetic products may be better, because the body doesn't react to them in the same way.

But best I found was desiccated thyroid extract by Armour. Desiccated (dried) thyroid is a thyroid hormone replacement drug, prepared from the thyroid gland from pigs -- also known as "porcine thyroid." Other brand names include Nature-throid, and Westhroid.

It has been on the market and safely used for more than 100 years. When synthetic thyroxine was introduced, there was a great deal of baloney and marketing hype about how modern it was, compared to "old-fashioned" desiccated thyroid -- and many doctors switched patients over to the synthetic medication. When the patient went into a steep decline as a result, he or she was told "It's your age."

All along, Synthroid has been sponsor of medical meetings, golf outings, symposia, research grants, and speakers' fees, and is the chief provider of lunches at medical offices, patient literature, pens, pads, mugs, and other freebies, giveaways, and marketing items for decades.

We now have several generations of doctors who have been trained to believe that synthetic levothyroxine -- and specifically Synthroid -- is the only thyroid replacement medication available or worth using. They simply don't know anything else. They hear ridiculous rumors on a regular basis -- spread by drug reps for competitive levothyroxine drugs -- that desiccated thyroid is going off the market.

Pseudo-Science

Most doctors claim their opposition to desiccated thyroid is science-based. However, that's not true, because there are no double-blind, peer-reviewed, double-blind studies that compare levothyroxine to desiccated thyroid in terms of effectiveness at resolving patient symptoms. So despite orthodox claims to rely on science, the fact is, the science doesn't exist to bolster the arguments that levothyroxine is superior to desiccated thyroid in resolving symptoms.

But things have got worse: much worse. Today, the profession has such an obsession with blood tests and lab work—and such a total belief in their accuracy and supremacy, that it has become considered quackery to ignore them. A doctor who administers thyroid supplements to a patient, when the blood tests are "normal" faces censure and loss of the right to practice medicine.

To treat a patient properly with clinical severe hypothyroidism may be as much as a physician's license is worth. To diagnose by the signs of the disease (the only reliable diagnostic method) is a lost art and patients face having it put down to aging and inadequacy. Some patients are even taken off thyroid replacement therapy because they "don't need it any more"; the blood tests have normalized.

So the poor patient's worthwhile life is ended, crucified on the cross of stupid and ignorant dogma. He or she declines in energy, looks, vitality, joy and sexuality. Weight gain is relentless; cholesterol soars; a heart attack becomes almost inevitable.

The trouble is that patients who are hypothyroid every often have normal levels of thyroid hormones, such as T4, T3 and the infamous TSH. The latter is taken as the absolute benchmark of thyroid performance. If it is normal, you don't have hypothyroidism.

Yet this situation (which is very common indeed) has parallels with diabetes type II, in which there is plenty of insulin—actually an excess—yet the body is not responding to it. What difference does it make if the body's thyroid hormone levels are "normal", if the cells in the tissues cannot respond to it?

High levels are even an indicator that the body is secreting excess hormone, to try and drive the cells, which are not actually responding.

Suppliers

You'll see Armour by Forest Labs, the oldest on the market, then Naturethroid and Westhroid which came into the picture in the late 1930's–by RLC Labs.

A new generic by Acella, NP Thyroid, hit the picture by late 2010 and is popular. There is Thyroid-S or "Thiroyd" from Thailand with excellent results, and Erfa's Thyroid from Canada. Australia uses compounded desiccated thyroid powder and there are many compounding (traditional) pharmacies around the world, which can help you.

It is always wise to start on a smaller dose of desiccated thyroid than they will ultimately need, such as 1 grain (60 mg). This will help the body improve and there may be other issues which can reveal themselves, such as sluggish adrenals or low Ferritin/iron levels.

But you will need to raise the dose quite soon, otherwise hypothyroid symptoms can return, due to the internal feedback loop in your body, which can happen if you stay on a low dose too long. Go to 2 grains in 2 – 3 weeks. Then 3 grains for a further 4 weeks, to give the T4 time to build (which can take 4-6 weeks). It's unlikely indeed that anyone would need more than 5 grains.

You can just swallow the grains or take them sublingually. When taking desiccated thyroid extract, it is important to avoid iron, estrogen and calcium supplements at the same time, since all bind the thyroid hormones to some degree.

Iron is important in this context: having low iron levels decreases deiodinase activity, i.e. it slows down the conversion of T4 to T3. Biologically, insufficient iron levels may be affecting the first two of three steps of thyroid hormone synthesis by reducing the activity of the enzyme "thyroid peroxidase", which is dependent on iron. Thyroid peroxidaxe brings about the chemical reactions of adding iodine to tyrosine (amino acid), which then produces T4 and T3.

Insufficient iron levels alter and reduce the conversion of T4 to T3, besides binding T3. Additionally, low iron levels can increase circulating concentrations of TSH (thyroid stimulating hormone).

You are looking for the removal of your hypothyroid symptoms, an afternoon temp of 98.6, a morning before-rising temp of 97.8 – 98.2 (held under arm ten minutes), good heart rate and blood pressure, good energy, clearing of brain fog, etc. We also found out that when optimal, our free T3 is at the top of the range, and free T4 is midrange. Note: if your free T3 is at the top of the range and you still feel horrible, time to test your iron (with blood) and cortisol levels (via saliva, NOT blood). Problems with either will cause T3 to pool high in your blood and not your cells.

Warning: This is not really a go-it-alone area for self-help. You need your blood levels monitored. Thyroid hormone is potentially harmful, even dangerous, and you would be wise to seek out a qualified medical practitioner of the open-minded sort, who can help and steer you.

Good website for self-help information and notes:
www.stopthethyroidmadness.com, run by Janie Bowthorpe. She knows more than me! (She should, she suffered thyroid Hell herself and has made a career out of learning the full thyroid story).

17 | Electromagnetic Energy Devices That May Help Prevent Aging

Pulsed Electromagnetic Devices For Extra Longevity
Nikola Tesla was the first modern individual to be recognized for manipulating electromagnetic fields for health purposes. His methods and patents in the early 1900s for the Tesla coil were also used for electromagnetic medical devices. [1]

These devices were often large round solenoid coils of wire that would surround the patient while they would stand or lie on a bed. They were energized directly from the 50 or 60 Hz sine wave electrical system. The patient would usually experience an immediate relief in pain.

Tesla's methods for electrotherapy were originally embraced by electricians who wanted to commercialize electricity. However electro-therapeutic devices eventually fell out of favor with doctors when educators in western medical schools chose to only educate medical students in the use of pharmaceuticals and surgery (a result of the infamous Flexner Report 1910).

In addition, a concerted effort by the pharmaceutical industry to discredit electromagnetic therapy caused it to be branded as "quackery" and electrical medical devices were only to be considered for diagnostic purposes such as X-ray. Tesla's advances were quickly forgotten.

The same could be said of the work of Georges Lakhovsky and his multiwave oscillator (MWO). By the 1920s, Lakhovsky had clinics all over Europe, delivering his electromagnetic oscillatory, or "vibrational" therapy.

Lakhovsky's method was so successful he was approached by several hospitals in New York hoping to test his apparatus experimentally. Remarkable results were obtained from a seven-week clinical trial performed at a major New York City hospital and that of a prominent Brooklyn urologist in the summer of 1941. What seemed like a promising development in the use of the MWO in America quickly faded after Lakhovsky unexpectedly died in New York in 1942 (age 73). *A car struck and killed him in a most mysterious manner.* His equipment was removed from the hospital and patients were told that the therapy was no longer available.

The murderous hand of Maurice Fishbein (the AMA) and Big Pharma is all over this story. The pharmaceutical companies and doctors figured out they could make a lot of money "treating" people, not making them well, and then getting someone else to pay for it. They continue to ruthlessly discredit valuable therapies that threaten their profits.

However, in the countries not under the sway of Big Pharma, like the former Soviet Union, electromagnetic field therapy did not die out, but was further developed and is still widely deployed throughout hospitals. Their scientists learned that when magnetic fields are pulsed, their effect was considerably enhanced. It covered the innate vibration of a wider range of cells and tissues, Lakhovsky would probably have said.

Pulsed Electromagnetic Fields (PEMF) was thus born.

Lower frequencies, that is frequencies below the commercial supply of 50 Hz (60 Hz in the USA) were found to be more biologically effective. I have already pointed out the work of others (including Robert Becker) in my book "Virtual Medicine", showing that these extremely low frequencies, or ELFs for short, have higher biological impact and that in the same way less intense fields are more effective biologically (not a case of "more is better").

With the fall of the Soviet Union, commercial enterprise was now possible with the West, allowing government controlled medical device manufacturers the authority to license their PEMF technology to neighboring countries such as Switzerland, Liechtenstein and Austria who eventually miniaturized and commercialized their products for hospital and home consumer use.

Although electromagnetic therapy has become widely adopted in Western Europe, its use was restricted to animals in North America. Veterinarians became the first health professionals to use PEMF therapy, for healing things like broken legs in race horses. Professional sports doctors then decided to experiment with veterinarian devices off label on professional athletes which ultimately led to legally licensed devices for human use in the United States - but under strict stipulations that it was not to be used for non-union bone fractures, except under a medical prescription from a licensed doctor.

Based on a 2007 clinical trial, Thomas et al. conclude, "PEMF may be a novel, safe and effective therapeutic tool." [2]

General Health Benefits
The whole of my book "Virtual Medicine" is about the existence of thrilling life energies, which inform and empower our cells and tissues. Atoms, molecules, cells and organs, all have different and unique characteristic oscillatory rates. Indeed, that is why cyclotron resonance devices (and dowsers) can detect specific tissues and disease processes.

Lakhovsky tells us that not only do all living cells produce and radiate their own oscillations, but they also receive and respond to oscillations imposed upon them from outside sources. Indeed, that's why cell phones, microwave radiation and so forth, is so inherently dangerous.

But why not give the cells a dose of healthy, "juicing up" vibrations, the sort that living organisms benefit from? Typically these are low frequency oscillations of ELFs, as they are called (extremely low frequencies). It is possible to enliven body tissues and healthy physiological mechanisms and structures by using pulsed electromagnetic fields.

A lot of people have caught onto this idea and it's working out just fine in practice, with or without the approval of regulatory bodies. As usual, where in one territory you are told it's illegal and maybe even dangerous, in other parts of the world it's everyday medicine from properly trained, certified and competent MDs and practitioners.

Wherever you live, you need to know about this up-and-coming therapy.

PEMF To The Rescue

This very week, my friend Marcus Freudenmann shared with me some research work done on the Continent. He and I just ran a cancer education conference together in London, with Colin Tipping and Dr. Med. Henning Saupe also contributing (2013).

Back at Dr. Saupe's clinic, in Kassel, Germany, a cancer patient was driven through the PEMF protocol, while Marcus and his sons watched and documented it all on film. What took place was remarkable, not just as a treatment for a cancer patient but for anyone, in any state of health. Especially, I would laud it as a treatment against any sort of aging, decay, metabolic slowdown or vascular insufficiency (the last covers most things due to aging!)

A sample of blood was taken and examined under dark field microscopy (which allows you to see living blood, instead of dead and stained specimens). What you see (image 1) is lots of red blood cells, stuck and jammed together in strings called "rouleaux" (like a pile of coins on its side). This is a bad formation that signifies sickness and means that red blood cells cannot flow freely through tiny capillaries and so deliver their "load" of oxygen efficiently. The blood is sludged, to use an everyday word.

Also, (arrowed) you will see a slightly different cell; that's a white blood cell. But it's quite as small as the red blood cells (it should be much larger, double or treble the size) and it is also very hemmed in and can't function.

Finally, pathology number three, if you look closely you will see the blood plasma, the background fluid, is filled with fibers, rather like carpet shedding its pile. That's *very* bad; those are fibrinogen threads and when present in large quantities like this acts like a buried mine that will explode at the least thing and cause instant clotting.

The more fibrinogen is present in the blood, the more likely a coronary thrombosis (myocardial infarction) or a stroke. Meantime, the fibers too add to the bloods overall viscosity or sludging. The rule is: the less viscosity, the better (providing the clotting mechanism is intact).

This sluggish blood was reflected in the patient, who said she was tired and had no energy.

It's important to remember that no chemical substance (vitamin C, DCA, B17, or Artemisin) which would normally be used for treatment of cancer would have any effect in such a state. Not even Otto Warburg's oxygen in high concentration could bind to these cells and mobilize the blood!

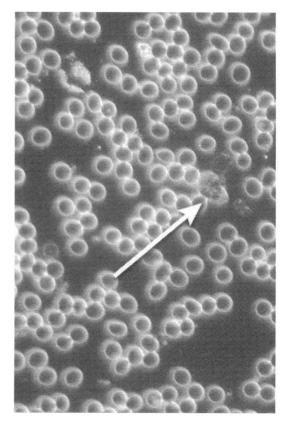

What followed was 15 minutes of PEMF therapy, directed towards her pelvis, chest, thyroid, pancreas and liver. And then another blood sample was taken (image 2). The changes that are evident are just amazing.

In such a short time the red cells have separated and are flowing smoothly and sweetly. When they bump into each other, they soon separate; in other words they do not stick together.

Also, the white cell is no longer trapped but disengaged and, most remarkable of all, it's more than doubled in size! Plus you can't see the fibers any more; the blood plasma is swept "clean".

This is of enormous importance to cancer patients, those fighting virtually any disease and those who resist aging. As Georges Lakhovsky taught us, our life is the energy in our cells. They vibrate and if that oscillatory rate drops to the levels shown by this lady, then blood perfusion drops and cancer is almost inevitable. Conversely, if we energize our cells with this kind of energy medicine treatment, the cells regain their gusto, move around and function as they should. Wow!

This is not to call it a cancer "cure". Indeed, it is different from many alternative therapies in that it is not aimed at the cancer at all; it's aimed at the blood support system and general cellular energies. Nevertheless, if you have fully understood what I have written here, you will likely judge this to be a must-have approach, in addition to anything else you may be employing, against your cancer (and, yes, even in conjunction with chemotherapy and radiotherapy).

Personally, I relish this against aging. As a confirmed "Boomer", I want to live a lot longer; the party we've always promised ourselves has only just begun! With PEMF to jolly up my tissues and keep them clean and refreshed, I expect to go on dancing a lot longer yet. Care to join me?

References:
1. Markov, Marko S. "Expanding Use of Pulsed Electromagnetic Field Therapies." Electromagnetic Biology & Medicine 26.3 (2007): 257–274. Academic Search Complete. EBSCO. Web. 10 June 2010.

2. Thomas, AW; Graham, K; Prato, FS; McKay, J; Forster, PM; Moulin, DE; Chari, S (2007). "A randomized, double-blind, placebo-controlled clinical trial using a low-frequency magnetic field in the treatment of musculoskeletal chronic pain". Pain research & management : the journal of the Canadian Pain Society = journal de la societe canadienne pour le traitement de la douleur 12 (4): 249–58.

Let There Be Light!

There is little doubt that the universe started as light. It happens to have emerged as one of the most potent properties of life. In a sense, we are light! That's not a New Age claim; that's scientific fact. Biophotons are here to stay.

Light is just part of the electromagnetic spectrum and we in turn are composed of electromagnetic energies. Energy, heat and light all come from this spectrum; today, every schoolkid knows that matter and energy are interchangeable. Voila! Light is life.

It has always been curious to me that the whole of the electromagnetic spectrum is hostile to biological life... except light and heat (and even heat can be damaging to life).

But not light!

Specifically, the band of waves that we call visible light. Once into the shorter wavelengths we call "ultraviolet", then it's not friendly at all. But then it's not light either, in the sense I am using it. The very name "ultra' violet means *beyond* visible violet light.

Small wonder then that light, used in the proper way, is very therapeutic. The Egyptians and Ancient Greeks knew it; they worshipped the Sun God: Amun (Amun-Ra) and Helios, respectively. Their temples were considered very healing.

Those of you who have read my book Virtual Medicine, will know I introduced several amazing light-based healing therapies. Light really is powerful stuff. Even the blind can get healed by light; how wonderful is that?

Seeing Red

One of the most fascinating breakthroughs in recent times has been the emergence of the healing powers of a specific band of red laser light (wavelength: 632.8 nanometres or often just sloppily stated as 635 nm). It rose to prominence in China and Russia, where is has been extensively studied and used therapeutically. Needless to say, Western medicine ignores it disdainfully.

Meanwhile, the science has started to roll in.

In one paper published in 2012, researchers evaluated 90 subjects. All of them had either coronary artery disease or a history of stroke. They divided the participants into a treatment group of 60 and a control group of 30. They gave the treatment group low level laser red light for just 30 minutes daily for 10 days, three days off and another session of 10 days. They exposed the control group to a normal, non-healing light.

The age range of the treatment and control group was similar (older demographic). The researchers evaluated their blood for blood viscosity and lipid changes. The two key blood viscosity measurements decreased significantly. That means their blood became less "thick" and easier to flow. That's extremely important for vascular diseases and also the ability to clean up the tissues and "detox".

Blood fats improved too. Total cholesterol fell from 173 mg/dl to 147. LDL fell from 107 mg/dl to 97 ;"good" HDL cholesterol rose from 42 mg/dl to 47; and, triglycerides (bad) fell from 161 mg/dl to 151.

Red light can help stroke. A 2005 China study on 21 patients utilized the sophisticated SPECT scan, which actually determines blood flow to various areas of the brain. The therapeutic light improved brain perfusion on the treated side! Other studies showed improvement in stroke symptoms with this treatment.

In another study conducted in 2003, Dou et al randomly divided 60 patients who had suffered a stroke to the brain (cerebral infarction) and 36 patients with traumatic brain injury into 2 groups (total of 96 patients). 50 of these patients were treated with intranasal light therapy (low level laser) and 46 with intravenous low level laser blood irradiation. Both were treated once a day for 5 consecutive days, given a 2-day break and resumed for another 5 days, adding to a total of 12 days in the study.

They found that total cholesterol, LDL cholesterol, triglyceride levels, erythrocyte sedimentation rate and the hematocrit (red blood cell level) were significantly reduced. Fugi Meyer movement scale (assessment of motor recovery after a stroke) and Barthel index scores (measurement of a person's daily functioning specifically the activities of daily living and mobility) were significantly increased. The damaged areas of the brain were reduced in both groups.

There was also no significant difference in whether the patients were being treated with Intranasal Light Therapy or intravenous blood irradiation therapy. [1. Dou Z, Hu X, Zhu H (2003). The effects of two kinds of laser irradiation on patients with brain lesion. Chin J Phys Med Rehabil. 25(2): 86-88 (in Chinese).]

In another (admittedly small) study, red light therapy was shown to cut cosmetic surgery wound healing time by half or one third, according to the researchers. They treated one half of the body and used the opposite side as its own "control". Their conclusion was clear: "In all instances, the LED therapy-treated side was statistically significantly superior to the unirradiated control by a factor of two to three." [J Cosmet Laser Ther. 2006 Apr;8(1):39-42]

It even works for allergic rhinitis; go figure! In a double-blind placebo-controlled study reported in the *Annals of Allergy, Asthma and Immunology* in April 1997, 72% of those receiving the "medical light" showed marked improvement, compared to 24% in the placebo group. The improvements were confirmed endoscopically, in 70% and 3% of cases, respectively, meaning that most of the placebo group believed they felt better but actually didn't show any physical improvements. [Ann Allergy Asthma Immunol. 1997 Apr;78(4):399-406]

These devices have already benefitted Parkinson's disease patients, those with sleep disorder and there is talk it may help to release growth hormone, which would be very valuable.

Cytochrome Oxidase

Then, what triggered me writing this, was a paper on PubMed published only a few days earlier, answering a very important question for Boomers and the whole anti-aging movement. Red light can beat senility; it can enhance cognitive function meaning: you hang onto your marbles a lot longer! This is hot stuff!

The use of transcranial lasers and LEDs enhances cognitive function, by lighting up your mitochondria, which are the tiny organelles in our cells that are like engines: they take fuel and burn it to create energy!

The researchers' conclusion (the Departments of Psychology, Pharmacology and Toxicology, University of Texas at Austin and the Department of Neurology and Neurotherapeutics, University of Texas Southwestern Medical Center, Dallas) is transcranial brain stimulation with low-level light/laser therapy (LLLT) using the red-to-near-infrared wavelengths is able to modulate neurobiological function. Unlike microwaves and cell phones, it does this in a nondestructive and non-thermal manner.

Tissues are completely unharmed by the "radiation". It's only light, after all.

The paper speculated that the mechanism of action of LLLT is based on photon energy absorption by cytochrome oxidase, the terminal enzyme in the mitochondrial respiratory chain. Cytochrome oxidase has a key role in neuronal physiology, as it serves as an interface between oxidative energy metabolism and cell survival signaling pathways. Cytochrome oxidase is an ideal target for cognitive enhancement, as its expression reflects the changes in metabolic capacity underlying higher-order brain functions. [Biochem Pharmacol. 2013 Aug 15;86(4):447-57. doi: 10.1016/j.bcp.2013.06.012. Epub 2013 Jun 24]

What's important for us is that you can grow new nerve cells, renew and invigorate the ones you've got, improve your arteries structure and their function, diminish inflammation and turn on half asleep energy modules called mitochondria.

Does that sound like anti-aging goodness? Or it is just good?

It's something we should all be doing.

Red Light Right Up Your Nose

Now the great news is that it's been found that ordinary red light of the same wavelength is almost as good as laser light. So no worry about safety issues. No electrical power supply needed. That means it's possible to get a real therapeutic effect just using a low-intensity battery-powered device. These come cheap, so this is a therapeutic breakthrough!

Now for the really fun part! The best way to administer magic "light food" is to shine it up your snout! I'm not kidding; intranasal light, as it's really called, has several advantages:

1. It's easy to do yourself
2. There is a rich capillary blood supply in the nasal cavities (once the blood is treated, that gets all round the body)
3. The whole area is just millimetres away from the brain itself!

So intranasal red light power has arrived (see illustration). Scientific studies show that the nasal route gives just as good results as IV treatment.

Now you can buy one of these devices for just a hair under $300. They last more or less indefinitely and you should use them daily, or at least several times a week. If you work it out over say a 5-year period, that's less than 2 cents a day.

I'd say that's a pretty good bargain for helping your body stay energized and your thinking on a clearer plane, for possibly years longer than otherwise!

Far Infrared Light

There are other devices using far infrared, instead of visible light (longer wavelength of 810 nm, and some are pulsed at 10 Hz, which is believed to make them more efficacious. It's all explained in the paper on intranasal light therapy and brain stimulation.

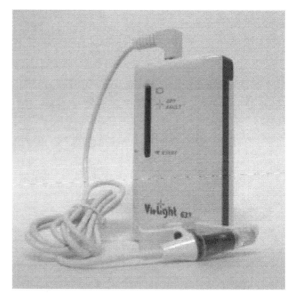

The pulsed mode of 10 Hz is most interesting. Based on studies with mice by Michael Hamblin of Harvard Medical School and other researchers, exposure to light at 810 nm and pulsing at 10 Hz, draws the greatest neurological healing in the brain that has suffered traumatic brain injury. This may be because of its closeness to alpha brainwaves frequency (when our brain is at rest or in meditative state) or in hippocampal theta state (which may help us with behavior inhibition). There is some claim of release of serotonin in this state, which would help in depression.

Using the wavelength of 810 nm gives deeper tissue penetration (reaching the deeper areas of the brain) without being outside the range that draws mitochondrial response. It just makes sense that this would help cover more areas of the brain, particularly the more ancient parts of the brain which happen to reside in the bottom sections and close to the nasal cavity. However, at this wavelength, the light is invisible to the naked eye – just be aware that the device is not broken, just invisible.

Light Helmets

This one is not quite ready for the market, as of the date of writing. But these devices will surely become available during the life of this edition of the book.

This too is not "red light" but near infrared. It can be supplied by helmets and were developed to help people with Alzheimer's disease make mental improvements. In some trials with senior citizens, it has actually fully reversed their Alzheimer's disease condition. Although this is a relatively new treatment for Alzheimer's the designer of the infrared light helmets named Dr. Gordon Dougal (a GP in the UK) has talked about the fact that these helmets promote neurogenesis in the brain as a result of treatment.

According to Dr. Dougal, these helmets work by directing intense bursts of infrared light into the brain to stimulate growth of brain cells. The reason he developed the helmet is because low-level infrared light is hypothesized to encourage brain cell growth and encourage tissue repair in the brain.

Allegedly, this infrared light helmet is able to reverse dementia symptoms like memory loss in just 30 days of treatment. Dementia sufferer Terry Pratchett (the writer) has had some success with the helmet and is helping to promote the concept.

The important point to grasp is the skull is not impenetrable to light but that, by shining infrared light onto a person's skin, the light goes into the frontal part of the brain as well as onto the side of the brain. The light penetrates brain tissue and is able to repair damaged tissue and help people grow new brain cells.

Your Personal Anti-Aging Program
(And My Good Health Wish For You)

You need to create for yourself some kind of self-determined anti-aging plan. It's just like any other goal in life: decide what you want, work out the steps to get it and then do those steps.

Here are a few thoughts from me, to help you do just that (not in any order of priority). You can change, extend or adapt this in any way you wish.

1. Create and Maintain a Healthy Mental Environment

Develop friends, clubs, family ties and hobbies. Be with people you like, doing stuff you like. It's crucial.

You also need to create yourself some nourishing goals. It's clear that people with a worthwhile purpose that carries them into the future will go on creating that future, as long as the inspiration lasts!

2. Track down your personal stressor foods and get off them. I can't stress enough that this is the number #1 anti-aging factor in the Universe!

3. Remove all manufactured foods from your diet and eat only whole foods. Reduce your carbohydrate intake to 100 gr. per day, maximum (2 slices of bread, 3 small potatoes). On no account eat refined carbohydrate, which means no sodas, ice cream, cookies, cakes or candy.

4. Make up your mind to do three 40-minute brisk walks every week. Try to make one of them last over an hour. You need to get out of breath and sweat by the finish. This is not time wasted; you'll get it back in useful years, later in your life. That's a promise.

5. Develop and strengthen your mind. Nothing gives more certainty of a healthy future than being able to project it in your thoughts. If you stay active and purposeful, with things to do that you enjoy, you WILL live beyond average. Read books, do crosswords, learn a language. No mind-dumbing activities like watching TV.

6. Do calming exercizes. I recommend my own CD on autogenic training. Or you can do meditation. Autogenics is easier for Westerners and less fanciful in its descriptions.

7. If you are over 60 and haven't done it yet, get a saliva test for your hormone levels. Supplement cautiously with a view to raising those which are low. If you can, work in conjunction with a knowledgeable anti-aging doctor.

8. Women, get a bone density screening. It makes a good baseline. The number one factor which determines whether you will get osteoporosis in your later years is where you started out. If your bones are thin at age 40, they will be really thin at age 80.

9. Work yourself out a supplements program and be sure to include the following:

1. Omega-3s — 2 gr daily
2. CoenzymeQ10 — 200 mg daily
3. Selenium — 100 mcg daily
4. Acetyl-L-carnitine — 500 mg daily
5. Alpha-lipoic acid — 200 mg daily
6. Vitamin C — 2 gr daily
7. Vitamin D — 2,000 mg daily.

That's as well as a fair shot at the others.

10. Top yourself up with iodine and repeat this from time to time.

11. Have a parasite cleanse and repeat every 6 months (see my eBook "Absolutely Disgusting: How To Diagnose And Treat Parasites").

12. Get a heavy metal detox. Christopher Shade's Intestinal Metal detox is the one I recommend.

13. Do the thermal chamber depuration program at least once. More if you have been in contact with heavy pollutants (such as close to agriculture, pesticides, working in a chemical plant, etc.)

14. Change your cosmetics to less toxic brands than those from major "name" manufacturers. The dazzling colors and needs of cosmetics when you were younger can mellow out into a modest fixing up of your face and hair. The less you do, the better your health, frankly. Do what I say in this book and you'll recover some of your former healthy "glow"!

15. Find love, even if it's a non-sexual relationship. Love keeps us all alive because it's what it means to BE alive! Try to avoid the squabbles which break up relationships because you will need each other in later life. Single and divorced people don't live as long. I can't insist you have regular sex, even though it's very good for you. But if you are alone, or your partner is not up for fun and excitement, you can masturbate regularly, at least 2-3 times a week and don't be ashamed.

16. Take your basal temperature regularly (see page 215 for instructions). With any suspicion of low thyroid function, get it dealt with. Even a 30-year old person would feel very, very old with low thyroid function.

17. Consider getting yourself an intranasal red light device, for quenching inflammation, energizing your mitochondria and growing a steady supply of new brain cells (good investment!) Also get started with soothing and calming binaurals. My own set "Love, Gratitude and Forgiveness" would be a great start and could give you a whole new look on life, as well as mitigating stress in your environment.

18. Sleep is crucial. If you are an insomniac get if fixed! Good sleep habits are among the most critical factors in successful aging.

19. Take your place proudly among the new "tribal elders" as you grow older and be proud of your life and achievements. You have knowledge beyond price, which is experience in life. Wear what you have learned with a grace and beauty and people will love you for it. Insist that people respect ancestors. We will all be ancestors some day.

20. Finally, stay current. This field is changing very swiftly. Try to keep connected with me, since I won't be giving you the hype and baloney from magazines or TV. Just the facts!

Made in the USA
San Bernardino, CA
30 June 2016